Women's Edge
HEALTH ENHANCEMENT GUIDE™

Get Well, Stay Well

*Your Complete Guide
to Achieving Optimum Health*

By Gale Maleskey, Deanna Portz, and the Editors of

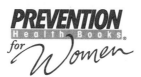

RODALE

© 2000 by Rodale Inc.
Illustrations © 2000 by Shawn Banner, Judy Newhouse, and Tom Ward

Printed in the United States of America on acid-free ∞, recycled paper ♲

Library of Congress Cataloging-in-Publication Data

Maleskey, Gale.
    Get well, stay well : your complete guide to achieving optimum health / by Gale Maleskey,
Deanna Portz, and the editors of Prevention Health Books for Women.
      p.   cm. — (Women's edge health enhancement guide)
    Includes index.
    ISBN 1–57954–239–5 hardcover
    1. Women—Health and hygiene.   2. Health.   3. Self-care, Health.   4. Consumer education.
I. Portz, Deanna.   II. Prevention Health Books for Women.   III. Title.   IV. Series.
RA778. M28 2000
613'.04244—dc21   00–036603

Distributed to the book trade by St. Martin's Press

2 4 6 8 10 9 7 5 3 1 hardcover

Visit us on the Web at www.rodalebooks.com, or call us toll-free at (800) 848-4735.

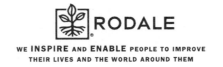

RODALE

WE **INSPIRE** AND **ENABLE** PEOPLE TO IMPROVE
THEIR LIVES AND THE WORLD AROUND THEM

Get Well, Stay Well Staff

EDITOR: E. A. Tremblay
ASSISTANT EDITOR: Debra L. Gordon
STAFF WRITERS: Gale Maleskey, Deanna Portz
CONTRIBUTING WRITERS: Julie Knipe Brown, Emily Dollemore, Leah Flickinger, Joely Johnson, Cheryl A. Romano, Elizabeth Shimer, Marie Elaina Suszynski
ART DIRECTOR: Darlene Schneck
COVER AND INTERIOR DESIGNER: Lynn N. Gano
ILLUSTRATORS: Shawn Banner, Judy Newhouse, Tom Ward
ASSISTANT RESEARCH MANAGER: Shea Zukowski
ASSISTANT FREELANCE RESEARCH MANAGER: Sandra Salera Lloyd
PRIMARY RESEARCH EDITOR: Anita C. Small
BOOK PROJECT RESEARCHER: Carol J. Gilmore
EDITORIAL RESEARCHERS: Molly Donaldson Brown, Grete Haentjens, Jennifer Bright Kaas, Jennifer S. Kushnier, Mary S. Mesaros, Valerie Rowe, Staci Ann Sander, Elizabeth Shimer, Lucille Uhlman, Teresa A. Yeykal, Nancy Zelko
SENIOR COPY EDITORS: Kathryn C. LeSage, Karen Neely
EDITORIAL PRODUCTION MANAGER: Marilyn Hauptly
LAYOUT DESIGNER: Donna G. Rossi
MANUFACTURING COORDINATORS: Brenda Miller, Jodi Schaffer, Patrick Smith

Rodale Healthy Living Books

VICE PRESIDENT AND PUBLISHER: Brian Carnahan
EDITORIAL DIRECTOR, *PREVENTION* GROUP: Anne Alexander
DIRECTOR OF NEW TITLE DEVELOPMENT: Tammerly Booth
DIRECTOR OF SERIES DEVELOPMENT: Gary Krebs
EDITORIAL DIRECTOR: Michael Ward
VICE PRESIDENT AND MARKETING DIRECTOR: Karen Arbegast
PRODUCT MARKETING DIRECTOR: Guy Maake
BOOK MANUFACTURING DIRECTOR: Helen Clogston
MANUFACTURING MANAGERS: Eileen Bauder, Mark Krahforst
RESEARCH MANAGER: Ann Gossy Yermish
COPY MANAGER: Lisa D. Andruscavage
PRODUCTION MANAGER: Robert V. Anderson Jr.
DIGITAL GROUP PROCESSING MANAGERS: Leslie M. Keefe, Thomas P. Aczel
OFFICE MANAGER: Jacqueline Dornblaser
OFFICE STAFF: Susan Dorschutz, Julie Kehs, Catherine E. Strouse

Prevention Health Books for Women Board of Advisors

Contents

**PART FOUR
A New
Beginning**

Introduction

There's no getting around it. However excellent our health, sooner or later, at some time in our lives, we all get sick. It's part of the human condition. And there's nothing like illness for making us feel totally and completely vulnerable.

As women, we're especially prone to feel that way, and with good reason: Many illnesses, like breast cancer, osteoporosis, and lupus, seem to have a special affinity for the female body. And others, like endometriosis, belong to us exclusively. To make matters worse, we're more sensitive to chemicals and toxins, like alcohol and cigarette smoke, than men are.

But that doesn't mean we're helpless. We don't have to be at the mercy of every microbe that happens to float by or every wayward gene that has set up shop in our cellular soup. We can defend ourselves. We can arm ourselves with knowledge, and with that knowledge come choices.

That's what this book is all about: choice and empowerment. It offers strategies for preventing disease and ways to fight it once it arrives. It will tell you how to identify signs and symptoms, and it will help you decide when to go for treatment as well as how to make sure that you'll get the very best of care.

You'll not only learn what to expect by way of diagnosis and treatment for individual ailments, you'll also explore the feelings women go through as they work their way back to health or accept the inevitability of a lifetime of coping.

Like every volume in the *Women's Edge* series, this book offers the very best natural options for prevention, care, and recovery from disease. But it will also show you which cutting-edge conventional medical treatments are available to you. You'll even find out why any symptom may be cause for attention but never for panic.

There is strength in wisdom. There is power in choice. This volume will give you both.

Anne Alexander
Editorial Director

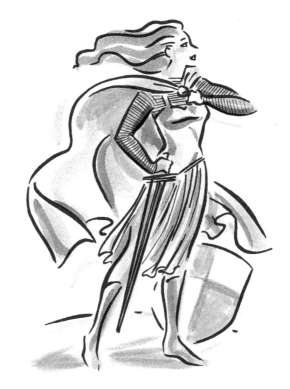

PART ONE

The Best Defense

Why We Get Sick

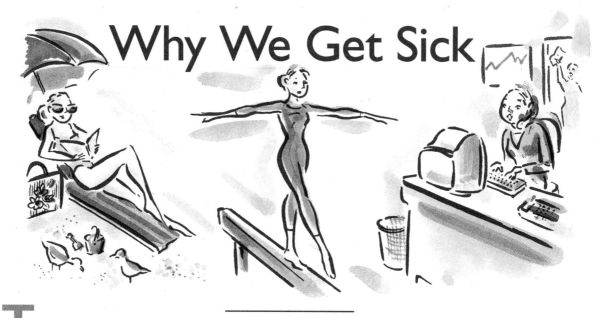

There's a word that describes a perfect state of balance: *equipoise*. It's a state we strive for in every aspect of our lives. We have families to care for, homes to maintain, careers to pursue, and personal needs to meet. We work, play, eat, and rest. And we try not to give any one part of our lives so much time, energy, or feeling that another part suffers. We're all aware of the pitfalls of putting career too much ahead of family or of all work and no play (it makes dull girls too). Balance is better.

Our health is the same way. The key to staying healthy is to keep all the aspects of our *selves*—the physical, emotional, and spiritual—in balance. When we do, we feel and function at our best. We're happy, creative, and productive. We have lots of energy, enjoy strong relationships, and are more able to handle the stressors in our lives. In short, we're healthy. Everything is in equipoise.

"Some people call it the zone," says Elaine Ferguson, M.D., a holistic physician practicing in Chicago and author of *Healing, Health, and Transformation*. "It's when you've reached the state where you're in harmony."

Illness, on the other hand, is a state of disharmony. We're functioning below our peak because some area of our health is out of balance, says Dr. Ferguson. Perhaps we have a serious illness such as cancer or a chronic disorder such as arthritis, or maybe we simply don't feel our best because of nagging headaches or fatigue.

"I see wellness and sickness as a continuum more than as distinct states," says Marcey Shapiro, M.D., a holistic physician practicing in Albany, California, who specializes in herbal medicine. At one end of the spectrum is optimal health, and at the other is serious illness. "Very few of us are at the extremes of having ideal health or being terribly ill," she says. "Most of us are somewhere in between."

Heeding the Signs

The symptoms we all get from time to time—stomachaches, insomnia, muscle tension—are warning signs that we're moving away from optimal health. We may not even be sick with a diagnosable illness, but our bodies are trying to tell us that something is out of balance, Dr. Ferguson says.

"We all have this intelligence within our bodies that speaks to us. The message could be a pain or a thought, but our bodies always tell us when something's wrong," Dr. Shapiro says.

It's our job to recognize these signs and pay attention to them. Heeding our bodies' signals will help us get back on the path to optimal health, but first we need to know what signals to watch out for. Here are the common physical, emotional, and mental symptoms that experts say can point to an imbalance in your health.

Muscle tension. Your muscles, especially in your neck, shoulder blades, and back, are full of tight knots.

Fatigue. Your energy level is so low that you just barely get through the day and then crash when you get home from work.

Loss of appetite. You don't feel hungry at mealtimes, and nothing seems appetizing to you.

Weight gain or weight loss. You've dropped or put on several pounds but haven't changed your eating or exercising habits.

Aches and pains. You have frequent, unexplained pain, such as headaches, stomachaches, or heartburn.

Difficulty sleeping. Several nights in a row, you have trouble falling or staying asleep.

MEDICINE THAT COMES IN PINK AND BLUE

"Sugar and spice, and everything nice, that's what little girls are made of. . . . Snips and snails, and puppy dog tails, that's what little boys are made of."

It's a nursery rhyme that speaks volumes. Scientists in the field of gender-based biology are now discovering that men and women actually are made of different stuff. "Women are not just small men," says Sherry Marts, Ph.D., scientific director of the Society for Women's Health Research, based in Washington, D.C. It turns out that men and women are different at the most basic level, the cellular level.

This discovery came about almost by accident. Researchers studying various drugs began noticing that some work better in women, while others are more effective in men. Take the over-the-counter drug ibuprofen, for example. When it comes to bringing down fevers and inflammation, ibuprofen works about the same in men and women. But it relieves pain much more effectively in men.

The differences don't end there. Diseases affect men and women in different ways as well. "Men tend to get diseases that are more urgent and tend to be more lethal. Women's diseases often start at a slower pace and cause disability long before death," explains Florence Haseltine, M.D., Ph.D., originator of the term *gender-based biology* and cofounder and former president of the Society for Women's Health Research.

By finding out why autoimmune diseases such as multiple sclerosis are much more common in women and why women develop heart disease decades later than men, we'll learn more about these diseases and develop better treatments for both women and men, Dr. Haseltine says.

As a result of these findings, someday doctors will treat the same disease differently, depending on the patient's sex, predicts Dr. Marts.

"It will translate itself almost immediately in the cardiac field," Dr. Haseltine says. "But I think the most exciting area of research is the study of structural differences in the brain and how brain disorders such as stroke are treated."

Hair loss. You notice more hair than usual in your brush or around the shower drain.

Dizziness or faintness. You feel weak and light-headed, especially when standing up. You may even have fainting spells.

Shortness of breath. You get winded when you walk to your car or up a flight of stairs.

Diarrhea or constipation. Your bowel movements are more frequent or less frequent than normal.

Anxiety. You feel tense and irritable and can't seem to escape your worries.

Disorganized thoughts. You have difficulty concentrating. You may lose things or forget appointments.

Depression. You are down in the dumps and feel hopeless.

Mood swings. Instead of being your typical pleasant self, you're moody and cranky much of the time.

"These are the signs that happen along the way when we move from optimal health toward illness," says Dr. Shapiro. "Usually, things start out as smaller signs that get louder and louder if people don't attend to them."

The problem is that it's easy to blame these symptoms on getting older or on the stresses of everyday life, so we end up dismissing them as quickly as they appear.

"We're so externally focused in terms of how we're taught to think and live that we don't pay attention to our bodies or our inner voices," Dr. Ferguson says. And the more we ignore our bodies, the further away we move from optimal health.

The good news is that we women have a built-in tool that helps keep us tuned in to our bodies. All we have to do is take advantage of it.

HAPPY TO BE HOSPITALIZED

We've all played hooky at least once in our lives—calling in to work sick when we barely had a sniffle. But some people practically make a career out of faking illness. They're sometimes called professional patients or hospital hobos by doctors because they travel from hospital to hospital claiming to be sick when, in fact, they don't have a physical illness at all. They have a mental disorder known as Munchausen syndrome.

The lives of people with this syndrome revolve around pretending to be sick. "They typically have poor relationships and spotty job histories," says Marc Feldman, M.D., an expert on Munchausen syndrome, an associate professor of psychiatry at the University of Alabama at Birmingham, and author of *Patient or Pretender*.

They lie about or exaggerate symptoms. Some even go so far as to make themselves sick. They may take poison, use their own feces to cause infections, and subject themselves to unnecessary surgery. If they're found out, they simply move on to another hospital in another city.

Often, they're seeking the attention, care, and concern that they lack in their lives, Dr. Feldman says. Or they may do it for the thrill of outsmarting highly trained, highly educated people. "Some patients describe it as an addiction, like gambling or alcoholism," he says.

How do they manage to dupe so many doctors? First of all, they play off doctors' expectations. "Physicians expect to

Women's Edge

Some women call it their intuition. Others say it's their sixth sense. Whatever you call it, women are more in touch with their bodies—and that gives them an edge over men when it comes to their health. "Men are taught from childhood to ignore pain rather than to stop and take care of it," says Royda Crose, Ph.D., associate director and associate professor of the Fisher Institute for Wellness and Gerontology at

see patients who are sick and want to be well—not patients who are well and want to be sick," Dr. Feldman says. Many of these people know a lot about the illnesses they fake. Some have worked in the medical field as receptionists or nurses. Others use the Internet to learn about the conditions they mimic. "The Internet has also given those with Munchausen syndrome a new forum," he says. They join on-line support groups and claim to suffer from chronic or incurable diseases, seeking warmth and support from the rest of the group.

Another form of this syndrome, called Munchausen by proxy, involves a parent faking or inducing illness in a child to gain "dutiful caregiver" status. Again, it's about getting attention as well as having some more complex needs met, says Judith Libow, Ph.D., coordinator of psychological services and training director in the department of psychology at Children's Hospital in Oakland, California. At least 95 percent of the time, the mother is the perpetrator, and it's estimated that 10 percent of these cases end in death, she says. A typical case involves a very young child who can't yet speak, a mother with an interest or training in health care, an uninvolved father, and a physician who becomes intensely involved in trying to solve the medical mystery.

"There are about three million reports of child abuse each year in this country. It would be wonderful to know how many of those involve Munchausen by proxy," Dr. Feldman says. "I receive an inquiry about Munchausen by proxy every day."

Ball State University in Muncie, Indiana, and author of *Why Women Live Longer Than Men.* Male professional athletes, for example, are notorious for playing while injured.

Women, on the other hand, are good at listening to their bodies. We're better listeners, in part, because the female body requires us to pay attention to its changes. "Our reproductive systems keep us tuned in to our bodies," Dr. Crose says. Because we menstruate, we learn at a young age that our bodies go through constant changes and that we feel physically and emotionally different throughout our cycles. Our periods are just the beginning. Our bodies make sure that we pay attention to them in many other ways as well.

When we get pregnant, for example, our bodies go through constant change for 9 months. During that time, we experience a part of being women that teaches us to be especially in tune with our physical well-being, Dr. Crose points out.

Even when we're not pregnant, most of us have annual gynecological exams and, after 40, mammograms. Eventually, of course, we also experience all the physical changes of menopause, such as hot flashes, mood swings, and the end of our monthly periods. "It's yet another time when our bodies go through changes and we become sensitive to everything that's going on inside of us," Dr. Crose says.

Call a Time-Out

Because all of these physical changes and trips to the doctor make us more aware of what's going on within our bodies, we're in a better position to recognize symptoms of illness when they crop up. But recognizing them isn't enough. We need to act. "When we notice signs that we're not feeling our best, we need to stop and take stock of our lives," Dr. Ferguson says. "I tell my patients to get very quiet and still and to listen and let their bodies tell them what they need to do."

We also need to question ourselves and our habits and examine the things that we've been doing, adds Heather Morgan, M.D., a holistic physician practicing in Centerville, Ohio.

REAL-LIFE SCENARIO

She's Running Herself Ragged and Getting Sick All the Time

Suzanna, 44, had it all: a beautiful home, an exciting job as a stockbroker, two daughters away at college, and a 25-year marriage. Then one night, her husband announced that he was divorcing her. Instead of caving in emotionally, Suzanna made him move out, then she threw herself into her work. She stayed at the office 12 hours a day, even on weekends. She didn't have time for breakfast or lunch—let alone time to think about the divorce. Soon, her body rebelled. She began feeling sluggish, then started getting frequent colds and headaches. She knows that she is wearing herself out but thinks that it's more important to get through this emotional crisis now and straighten out her health habits later. Is she right?

If Suzanna doesn't invest some time and effort into her physical and emotional health, she could be a stockbroker headed for a crash. Her headaches are no doubt a by-product of all this stress, and her weakened immune system is likely a result of stress and poor diet. She could be setting herself up for a serious illness, such as heart disease.

Suzanna is not taking care of herself emotionally either. It's perfectly normal for someone going through a divorce to be sad, angry, and scared. She should see a psychotherapist, who can help her face her feelings and teach her healthier ways to cope with stress.

Suzanna can also do some things on her own. She needs to make time for breakfast and lunch and start an exercise program. She'll relieve stress, increase her energy level, and improve her emotional well-being—all things that positively impact the immune system. Suzanna also needs to set aside some quiet time each day to connect with her feelings, perhaps through yoga or meditation. And above all, she has to get together with friends on the weekends instead of isolating herself at the office.

Expert consulted
Mary Claire Wise, M.D.
Holistic family physician
Rochester, New York

Any number of events can knock us off-kilter. Maybe we have picked up a virus, are grieving the loss of a loved one, or are questioning our spiritual beliefs, Dr. Ferguson says. Perhaps we are under a lot of stress, aren't getting enough sleep, or are routinely passing up nutritious food for high-fat fare. "Everything from our relationships and emotions to what we eat, breathe, and touch affects our health," she says. Our hormones, our expectations, and, of course, our genes all play a role.

So does the fact that we're women. "Scientists are just beginning to discover the enormous impact that our sex has on our health," says Sherry Marts, Ph.D., scientific director of the Society for Women's Health Research, based in Washington, D.C.

Beyond Having Babies

Our ability to bear children is not the only thing that makes us different from men. Being female has a great deal of influence over our health. "We're starting to see that there are definitely a lot of physiological differences between men and women," Dr. Marts says. Because our bodies are different than men's, various illnesses and treatments affect us differently as well, she says.

For example, women appear to be more susceptible than men to certain chemical substances, such as alcohol and the carcinogens in cigarettes. Research shows that women develop cirrhosis of the liver after a shorter period of heavy drinking than men do. Women also have a 20 to 70 percent higher risk of developing lung cancer than men at every level of exposure to cigarette smoke.

Women also suffer from certain diseases more often than men. About 75 percent of all people with autoimmune diseases, such as multiple sclerosis and lupus, are female.

When we do get sick, women experience symptoms that are different from men's for the same conditions. A man suffering a heart attack, for example, is likely to have gripping chest pain, while a woman is more likely to have subtle symptoms such as abdominal pain, nausea, and extreme fatigue.

Beyond symptoms, diseases may actually progress differently in men and women. Women with multiple sclerosis, for example, tend to experience periods of remission followed by relapses, while men with the disease tend to have continuously progressive symptoms. In addition, some research suggests that HIV-positive women progress to AIDS at a lower viral load than men, which means that women have less virus in their blood when they start to develop opportunistic infections and other symptoms of full-blown AIDS.

There are even differences between men and

MY MAMA TOLD ME

Can reading in dim light really ruin my eyes?

You may find reading in dim light hard to do, but it won't hurt your eyes. Moms probably tell their kids not to read in the dark because they have a tough time doing it themselves. It turns out that kids' eyes can gather more light, so children need less light to read than adults do.

If Susie likes reading with a flashlight under her blanket, there's no need for her to close the book. She can finish the story, and Mama can rest easy.

Expert consulted
Anne Sumers, M.D.
Ophthalmologist
Spokesperson for the American Academy of
*   Ophthalmology*
Ridgewood, New Jersey

women where treatment is concerned. Drugs are processed and handled differently in a woman's body and affect its systems differently. Ibuprofen, for example, is less effective at providing pain relief for women. Women also wake up from anesthesia an average of 4 minutes faster than men.

It all comes down to something most of us intuitively know: To prevent and heal illness, we not only need to listen to our bodies and keep ourselves in balance, we also have to establish health habits that address our special needs as women.

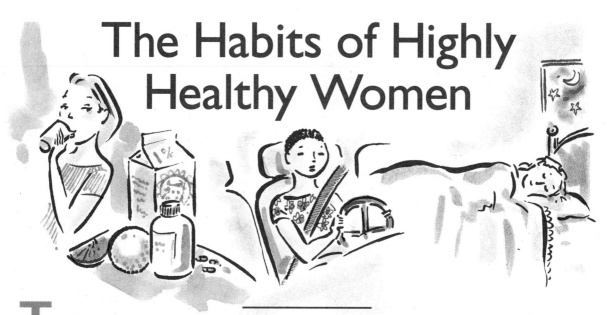

The Habits of Highly Healthy Women

T here is no animal more invincible than a woman," said poet and playwright Aristophanes. And in one way, he may have been right. Although men clearly have physical advantages over women in strength, height, and muscle tone, when it comes to longevity, there's no contest. According to documented mortality data, women have been outliving men since at least the 1500s, and these days we outlive them by an average of 5 years—life expectancies are 79 years for women and 74 years for men.

Our predisposition to live longer does not, however, mean that we can sit back at our leisure and enjoy better health with no effort. To gain from our biological advantages, we have to work at taking good care of ourselves. Here's a top 10 list of health habits we all should strive for.

1. Move Your Body

Exercise improves cardiovascular health, which helps prevent heart disease, high blood pressure, and diabetes, explains Sherry Marts, Ph.D., scientific director of the Society for Women's Health Research, based in Wash-

ington, D.C. It also helps you look better, have more energy, and be less likely to get depressed. To get the most mileage for your sweat, exercise both aerobically and with weights. "There is also some data showing that weight-bearing exercise prevents osteoporosis, particularly when it's done in your twenties and thirties," she says.

Get your heart pumping. "Walk, and walk faster," says Trudy L. Bush, Ph.D., professor of epidemiology and preventive medicine at the University of Maryland School of Medicine at Baltimore. "All you need is a pair of athletic shoes." For both your heart and your waistline, the American College of Sports Medicine recommends that you exercise aerobically at a moderate pace for 20 to 60 minutes a day 3 to 5 days a week.

Pump yourself up. "Resistance training, such as lifting weights, increases and maintains muscle and bone, which improves body composition and appearance and increases your metabolism," says Jennifer Layne, a certified strength and conditioning specialist and exercise physiologist at the Jean Mayer USDA Human Nutrition Research Center on Aging at Tufts

University in Boston. And resistance training builds your strength, which makes daily life activities easier. The American College of Sports Medicine recommends doing a routine, 2 or 3 days a week, consisting of 8 to 10 exercises that work the major muscle groups. Strive for 8 to 12 repetitions of each exercise.

2. Eat a Healthful, Diverse Diet

Eating a nutritious, varied diet helps lessen your risk of heart disease and certain cancers, such as colon cancer. "Eat lots of fiber, fruits, and vegetables, and a reasonable amount of fat," advises I-Min Lee, M.D., assistant professor of epidemiology at Harvard School of Public Health and assistant professor of medicine at Harvard Medical School. The American Heart Association (AHA) considers no more than 30 percent of daily calories to be a reasonable amount of fat, with less than 10 percent coming from the saturated fats contained in animal products. "It's also important to watch your total calorie intake," she says.

Get your fruits and veggies. The AHA recommends that you eat five or more servings of vegetables, fruits, or fruit juices a day. Fruits and vegetables pack lots of vitamins, minerals, and fiber without adding many calories. If fruits and vegetables sound boring—and let's face it, sometimes they are—Ann Gentry, chef and owner of the organic, vegetarian Real Food Daily Restaurant in Los Angeles, recommends that you boost their appeal by buying them fresh (preferably from a farmers' market) and by putting more thought into the way you arrange and serve them. "Think color and texture," says Gentry. Put three to five different-colored vegetables on a plate, and use bigger pieces, smaller pieces, and different cuts. A variety of colors also indicates a variety of nutrients.

Control your appetite for critters. The AHA recommends that you keep your daily intake of poultry, fish, or lean meat to no more than 6 ounces a day. If greasy ribs are your only passion at mealtimes, try using different meats, such as lean cuts of wild game, buffalo, or ostrich, and add flavor with some spices.

MY MAMA TOLD ME
Will going barefoot really give me flat feet?

Going barefoot may make your feet dirty, but it won't make them flat. Some people are born with the collapsed arches that give a person flat feet. Your arches can also collapse if you spend a lot of time on your feet but don't have adequate arch support in your shoes.

Your mom probably told you not to go barefoot outdoors because she knew of all the dangers. You could hurt your feet by stepping on glass or a rusty object. Hard surfaces like asphalt are hot and may be hard on your feet. If you have any heel pain or foot problems, walking on concrete or asphalt can aggravate the condition. What's more, if you go barefoot on wet surfaces, such as at a public pool or in community showers, you could pick up the microbial organisms that cause athlete's foot or painful plantar warts.

Expert consulted
Pamela Colman, D.P.M.
Director of health affairs
American Podiatric Medical Association
Bethesda, Maryland

WOMAN TO WOMAN

She Made Kicking the Habit a Family Affair

Longtime smoker Agatha Johnson-Page, 57, had tried to quit before, but hypnosis and stopping cold turkey didn't do the trick. Now, thanks to a popular drug and the support of her family, she has kicked the habit for good. Here's her story.

I had my first cigarette at age 16. My friends smoked, so I tried it—and before long, I was hooked. At that time, no one knew it was a health hazard.

I smoked half a pack a day for about 20 years. Then I quit cold turkey but started smoking again 6 months later when I needed a way to relieve stress.

Since then, I've tried to quit a number of times. I even went to a group hypnosis session where we all tossed our cigarettes in the trash as we left.

Finally, two of my kids and I quit together, and none of us has had a cigarette since June 1998. The support system we created really helped. We shared our success stories, encouraged each other, and called each other if we thought we might slip. Quitting with my kids also gave me an extra incentive: I didn't want to falter, because I didn't want them to falter.

My daughter used nicotine patches, and my son and I took the prescription drug Zyban. After the first week, I didn't get much pleasure out of smoking anymore. And now I can't stand being around cigarette smoke. I find it offensive.

I figured that at my age, after smoking for some 40 years, quitting wouldn't really improve my health. Boy, was I wrong. I always used to cough and blow my nose in the morning, but since I've quit smoking, I don't wake up congested anymore. I'm also able to hold my notes longer when I sing in my car. And I'm a much cleaner, healthier person.

I did gain a few pounds, but I didn't let that discourage me. I figure that's the next thing I'll work on.

Several of my friends still smoke, and at first I was worried I'd slip back into the habit when I was around them. But I just went on a 4-day trip with two of my friends, and I didn't have a single craving. That was my big test, and I aced it.

Expand your food horizons. You can find an endless number of tasty and healthful foods if you open up your mind along with your mouth. "To add more variety to your diet, add exotic vegetables like yams and winter squash, and experiment with spices," says Dr. Bush.

Basic spices can give food great flavor. "Use basil, oregano, thyme, rosemary, and cilantro," Gentry suggests. "And definitely put them on during the cooking." She also suggests cooking with miso, which is a soybean paste. "Whether you're making soups, pastes, sauces, or spreads, miso can really go a long way."

3. Bone Up on Calcium

Before the onset of the agricultural age 10,000 years ago, humans appear to have been high consumers of calcium. Nowadays, we probably eat only one-fourth to one-third the calcium that our ancestors did, and that's not enough. Osteoporosis affects 20 million American women, and one of the best ways to prevent the disease is with calcium. Here's how to boost your intake.

Dine on some dairy. "Eat yogurt and other calcium-rich foods," says Dr. Bush. The National Institutes of Health suggests that you get 1,000 to 1,500 milligrams of calcium daily. Try to choose nonfat or low-fat dairy products such as fat-free milk or low-fat cheese.

Supplement it. "Most Americans don't get enough calcium in their diets," says Dr. Lee. To up your intake, you can take supplements.

But keep your total daily intake from diet and supplements below 2,500 milligrams, says Lila A. Wallis, M.D., clinical professor of medicine at Weill Medical College of Cornell University in New York City and coauthor of *The Whole Woman*. Higher doses must be taken under medical supervision.

4. Get Enough Sleep

The quality of your Zzzs may determine not only your well-being the next day but also your physical health for years down the road. "Sleep deprivation may reduce your body's defenses and increase your risk of disease," says Dr. Lee. It's believed that when you fall asleep, infection-fighting blood cells move from your bloodstream into your tissues, attacking viruses and bacteria as you snooze.

Sleep deprivation can also affect your emotional well-being. You may be more testy, and your attention span may suffer, says Rosalind Cartwright, Ph.D., director of the Sleep Disorder Service and Research Center at Rush–Presbyterian–St. Luke's Medical Center in Chicago. Here are suggestions to help you improve your sleep patterns.

Replace lost hormones if you are postmenopausal. "Since the hormones we lose at menopause are implicated in the breathing disorders of sleep, supplementation is a

TOP 10 KILLERS OF WOMEN

Young Women (Ages 25 to 44)
1. Cancer
2. Accidents
3. Heart disease
4. AIDS
5. Suicide
6. Homicide
7. Stroke
8. Chronic liver disease and cirrhosis
9. Diabetes
10. Pneumonia and influenza

Middle-Aged Women (Ages 45 to 64)
1. Cancer
2. Heart disease
3. Stroke
4. Chronic obstructive pulmonary disease
5. Diabetes
6. Accidents
7. Chronic liver disease and cirrhosis
8. Pneumonia and influenza
9. Suicide
10. Blood infection

Senior Women (Ages 65 and Up)
1. Heart disease
2. Cancer
3. Stroke
4. Chronic obstructive pulmonary disease
5. Pneumonia and influenza
6. Diabetes
7. Accidents
8. Alzheimer's disease
9. Kidney disease
10. Blood infection

THE WORST HEALTH HABITS A WOMAN CAN HAVE

Unfortunately, not all of the choices we make regarding our health are good ones. In fact, when it comes to bad habits, these top the list.

Lighting up. Unless you've been in hiding for the last 30 years, you know that smoking is bad for you. In addition to being a major factor in heart disease, lung cancer, and stroke, smoking causes emphysema, skin wrinkling, and bone loss. But despite the repeated warnings, about 23 percent of all women still smoke.

Basking in the sun. About 80 percent of skin cancers are caused by sun exposure—a big price for a good tan. "Sunbathing also promotes wrinkling and dry skin," says Trudy L. Bush, Ph.D., professor of epidemiology and preventive medicine at the University of Maryland School of Medicine at Baltimore.

Hitting the sauce too hard. "Drinking large amounts of alcohol is definitely a no-no," says I-Min Lee, M.D., assistant professor of epidemiology at Harvard School of Public Health and assistant professor of medicine at Harvard Medical School. Overconsumption of alcohol has been linked to an increased risk of breast cancer and possibly to an increased risk of certain types of stroke. Small amounts are okay since alcohol lowers the risk of heart disease, she says. For optimum health, limit yourself to three to four drinks a week and no more than one drink in a day, says Dr. Bush.

Being a couch potato. A sedentary lifestyle puts you at risk for a long list of problems, such as heart disease, osteoporosis, obesity, and depression, says Lila A. Wallis, M.D., clinical professor of medicine at Weill Medical College of Cornell University in New York City and coauthor of *The Whole Woman*. Any type of motion that separates you from the sofa is better than none. For best results, Dr. Wallis suggests that you regularly engage in a repetitive activity that increases your breathing and heart rate.

Having bad eating habits. A diet high in saturated fat, sugar, and meat, and too low in vegetables and whole foods is likely to take a negative toll on your body, possibly leading to heart disease, cancer, and chronic gastrointestinal problems.

good idea," says Dr. Cartwright. "Hormone supplements also reduce sleep disturbances caused by hot flashes."

Stick to a regular schedule. "If you don't sleep long enough one night, don't go to bed earlier the next night," says Dr. Cartwright. Going to sleep and getting up at the same time every day will help establish a regular sleep/wake cycle.

Behave yourself before bedtime. Your activities immediately before you hit the sack can interfere with your sleep. "Avoid heavy meals or booze before bedtime," says Dr. Cartwright. Heavy meals could cause heartburn, and alcohol, although it makes you drowsy, will wake you up about 3 hours later. And although walking has been shown to promote good sleep, don't work out less than 4 hours before hitting the sack, because exercise's stimulating effects may up your sheep count.

If you must nap, keep it short. "If you need to extend your waking hours, a 15- to 20-minute nap midday will help," says Dr. Cartwright. "Longer naps make you wake up with a 'sleep hangover' and may interfere with your sleep that night."

5. Stop Stressing

"Stress results from the perception that you are ill-equipped to meet the demands on your mind and body," says Margaret Caudill, M.D., Ph.D., codirector of the department of pain medicine at Dartmouth-Hitchcock Medical Center in Manchester, New Hampshire. Stress can also result from an overload of positive activities, such as when planning a wedding. "Unchecked stress can cause decreased sleep, muscle tension, heart palpitations, shortness of breath, and irritable bowel symptoms," she says. Long-term stress may lead to the development of chronic health problems such as high blood pressure and decreased immune function. To help destress yourself, consider this advice.

Listen to your body. "It's important for people to identify their stress symptoms," says Dr. Caudill. Most of us know how we react to stress—your neck tenses up, your stomach hurts, you can't sleep, you suddenly have a headache, or you feel irritable. The key is to home in on the symptoms early so you can quickly take steps to deal with the stressful situation that's causing them.

Do something for yourself. If you're like many women, you nurture everyone else at the expense of satisfying your own needs. It helps to make a commitment to yourself, says Dr. Caudill. "Do something on a regular basis to relieve tension," she says. It doesn't take much—get some exercise or just take a few deep breaths.

Meditate. "Repeatedly focusing on a word, phrase, breath, or motion can cause the relaxation response during and after meditation, which can reduce stress-related changes in your body," says Dr. Caudill. Meditate once a day for 10 to 20 minutes to rejuvenate both your body and your mind.

6. Pay Your Doctor a Visit

Yearly exams can prevent a number of conditions, including breast and cervical cancers and osteoporosis, says Dr. Wallis. Have your body screened with these tests.

Get a mammogram. "The mortality rate from breast cancer is decreasing, which is prob-

ably related to the detection of early lesions by mammogram," says Paula Szypko, M.D., a pathologist at North State Pathology Associates in High Point, North Carolina, and spokesperson for the College of American Pathologists. Premalignant and early noninvasive tumors can be detected by a mammogram before they can be felt. Dr. Szypko suggests going for an annual mammogram every year after age 40. "In addition, do monthly self-examinations and have an annual examination by your health-care practitioner," she says.

Prevent cancer with a Pap test. "The death rate from uterine cervical cancers has dropped significantly since the Pap test became available almost 50 years ago. It went from being number one to not even being in the top 10," says Dr. Szypko. The preventive effects of the test are tremendous. Eighty percent of women who die of cervical cancer have not had a Pap test in 5 years. She recommends that you have an annual Pap test starting at age 18. "A lot of women believe that they don't need to have Pap tests if they're beyond their childbearing years, but 60 percent of cervical cancers occur in women over age 55," she says.

Give the rest of your body a once-over. In addition to a Pap test and mammogram, you should have an annual flu shot and cholesterol and blood pressure checks, says Dr. Bush. Women over 45 should have a dual-energy x-ray absorptiometry (DEXA) bone scan to check for osteoporosis. If you're over 50, you should also undergo a screening for rectal and colon cancers every 5 to 10 years.

7. Buckle Up

"I'm only going a few blocks." "I don't want to wrinkle my dress." The list of excuses goes on. But every hour, somebody dies as a result of failure to wear a seat belt. And if the threat to

WHY WOMEN LIVE LONGER THAN MEN

It's been documented for hundreds of years and known for thousands: Women live longer than men. But why? Here are some possibilities suggested by Royda Crose, Ph.D., associate director and associate professor of the Fisher Institute for Wellness and Gerontology at Ball State University in Muncie, Indiana, and author of *Why Women Live Longer Than Men*.

Testosterone is troublesome. "Testosterone seems to be related to increased activity, impulsiveness, and aggressiveness, which can lead to risky behavior," says Dr. Crose. In their younger years, men are more likely than women to die from accidents, suicide, and homicide. Later in life, testosterone increases bad low-density lipoprotein cholesterol and decreases good high-density lipoproteins, putting men at a greater risk for heart disease.

Estrogen protects. "Medical scientists believe that premenopausal women enjoy a buffering effect from illness, because of estrogen," says Dr. Crose. Estrogen is believed to protect women against heart disease, osteoporosis, and possibly brain disorders such as Alzheimer's disease.

Illness gets crossed out. "Scientists believe that females have an advantage in having two X chromosomes, because the second X chromosome provides a backup if something goes wrong with a gene on the first one," says Dr. Crose.

Pears are healthier than apples. Women typically gain weight in their lower bodies—their hips, buttocks, and legs—giving them more of a pear shape, while men are more apple-shaped. "The apple-shaped pattern of obesity is believed to be a strong predictor of increased high blood pressure, diabetes, heart disease, and stroke," says Dr. Crose.

If you still absolutely refuse to buckle up when you're driving alone, at least buckle up in front of your children. If you don't, you send a message that it's okay to go without a seat belt. The American College of Emergency Physicians (ACEP) reports that when a driver is not wearing a seat belt, young passengers will only be buckled 30 percent of the time, versus 94 percent of buckled drivers' young passengers.

And remember that *all* passengers should buckle up. The ACEP states that in a 55-mile-per-hour crash, an unrestrained backseat passenger could fly forward at a force strong enough to seriously injure or even kill a person in the front. So for your own safety and that of your fellow passengers, make sure that everyone is belted.

Finally, make sure that you're buckled properly. According to the AAA, a seat belt worn incorrectly could do more harm than good. The belt should be over your hips and pelvis, in front of your chest, and over your shoulder. A belt worn behind your body could cause your head to hit the dashboard, and a belt worn under your arm could break your ribs and lead to serious internal injuries.

your life won't convince you, maybe the threat to your wallet will. A primary seat-belt law in 16 states and the District of Columbia allows a police officer to pull you over and cite you specifically for not buckling up. There's really no excuse for not spending the 3 to 7 seconds it takes to fasten your seat belt.

8. Renew Your Relationships

"People who are emotionally connected to other people do better in terms of disease risk than people who are not connected," says Dr. Lee. The effects of isolation are even worse for people with chronic illness. People with coronary artery disease who have spouses or confidantes, for example, are 30 percent more likely to survive than patients who are isolated. "Whether it's church, your partner, or your friend, just having support helps," she says. Here are a few ways you can stay connected.

Build a support network. "People with good social health have relationships that are interdependent and complementary, where each person helps the other," says Royda Crose, Ph.D., associate director and associate professor of the Fisher Institute for Wellness and Gerontology at Ball State University in Muncie, Indiana, and author of *Why Women Live Longer Than Men.* "Such interdependent relationships provide a safety net that's important for survival throughout life but is especially crucial in old age."

Keep your love alive. To remain zestful, love relationships need a constant supply of fresh energy. Be spontaneous with your partner, whether you make a last-minute decision to walk in the park or to fly to the Bahamas. And remember to laugh—it boosts the joyful spirit that connected you in the first place, says Dr. Crose.

Explore your spirituality. Religious activities can give meaning to your life and provide personal satisfaction outside your family. "Spiritual and religious connections provide motivation and hope—outlooks that promote longevity," says Dr. Crose.

9. Laugh Out Loud

Laughter is the physiological response to humor. Research suggests that laughter produces physiological benefits, including increased antibodies, decreased stress hormones, and a higher pain threshold. "Laughter is also good for your emotional health," says Dr. Bush.

According to a study done at Loma Linda University in California, when heart attack patients added a 30-minute humorous video to their cardiac rehabilitation, they had lower blood pressure, fewer stress hormones, and lower medication requirements.

10. Have a Hobby

"Women spend too much time doing things for others," says Dr. Bush. Doing an activity for your own sake provides a source of enjoyment that can reduce stress and improve well-being, she says. To incorporate a new activity into your life, try the following.

Look back to your youth. "Renew a hobby you had earlier in life," suggests Dr. Bush. Whether it's painting, playing cards, or even mall walking, if you enjoyed it before, take it up again.

Dig in the dirt. Gardening is an excellent hobby, says Dr. Bush. Garden work has been shown to spark creativity and optimism, and physically, it burns calories and can lower blood pressure.

Volunteer. "I think that volunteering, the idea of altruism, is important," says Dr. Caudill. "It's been demonstrated that people who make connections with people and do things for others are healthier."

By volunteering, you can enhance your own life as you learn new skills and form new relationships, says Dr. Crose.

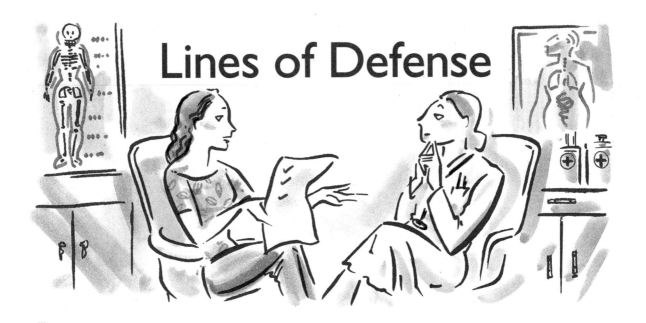

Lines of Defense

If it's true that an apple a day keeps the doctor away, we must be eating an awful lot of apples, because our doctors aren't spending much time with us at all. In fact, a typical primary-care physician spends less than 13 minutes with each patient every 6 months.

That doesn't leave much time for the kind of basic preventive medicine that can help to keep us healthy. In a 1998 survey conducted by the Commonwealth Fund, only 55 percent of women reported that their blood cholesterol had been tested in the previous year. Nearly 40 percent said that they had not had physical exams or Pap tests. One in three had not undergone clinical breast exams. And one in six had not received any preventive care during that time.

But time is not the only problem. A lack of incentives—doctors aren't compensated by insurers for most types of preventive care—also tends to discourage physicians from suggesting precautionary measures that would have long-term impact on women's health, points out Linda Hyder Ferry, M.D., associate professor of preventive medicine and family medicine at Loma Linda University School of Medicine in California. In addition, many doctors simply haven't been adequately trained in preventive care.

"Physicians traditionally are not taught how to be good prevention counselors," Dr. Ferry says. "I did my own survey of every medical school in the United States. The survey asked about the training available concerning tobacco. The results were discouraging. Tobacco use is the leading preventable cause of death in the United States, yet most medical schools do not require clinical training in helping patients to stop smoking. Nutritional training is even worse."

So, like it or not, the burden of responsibility for preventive care rests primarily on our own shoulders.

"Women must become consumer advocates for themselves. They need to read everything they can about preventive care because most physicians, unless they have taken time on their own to learn about these issues, aren't likely to provide the best prevention strategies," Dr. Ferry says.

Eat Good Food to Sidetrack Ailments

The USDA Food Guide Pyramid is an excellent foundation for helping people prevent many illnesses, says Jennifer Brett, N.D., a naturopathic physician in Stratford, Connecticut. The pyramid says that women should eat 6 to 11 servings daily of bread, cereal, rice, and pasta; 2 to 4 servings of fruits, such as apples, strawberries, and bananas; 3 to 5 servings of vegetables, such as broccoli, tomatoes, and lettuce; 2 to 3 servings of milk, yogurt, cheese, and other dairy products; and 2 to 3 servings of meat, poultry, fish, dried beans, eggs, or nuts. Fats should be used sparingly. But the pyramid is just one of many tools that women should use to maintain their health.

"Your entire health derives from what you do every day. All the pills in the world aren't going to make up for a bad foundation. So you have to start off with balanced nutrition," Dr. Brett says. "Of course, there are specific needs for individuals that must also be accounted for. A woman with recurring yeast infections, for instance, might help herself prevent those infections if she eats foods that contain less sugar, starch, and other refined carbohydrates."

Although every woman's dietary needs differ slightly, here are a few general guidelines that, in addition to the food pyramid, can help keep you in peak nutritional condition.

BETTER FOODS FOR BETTER HEALTH

Eating more organic, natural products can help you maintain your health, says Jennifer Brett, N.D., a naturopathic physician in Stratford, Connecticut. Many commercial products on a typical grocery shelf these days contain chemicals, hormones, and other unnatural additives that can trigger food allergies and compromise your overall health. Naturally grown staples and other organic products are available at most health food stores. For starters, consider adding the following natural foods to your shopping list.

- Amaranth. It is a near-complete protein, loaded with calcium and other vital nutrients. It's available as a seed, as flour, or puffed.
- Arrowroot. Instead of cornstarch, which may cause constipation, diarrhea, and vitamin loss, use arrowroot as a thickening agent in recipes. Arrowroot also has less of an aftertaste than cornstarch. For people who are allergic to corn, it is a perfect substitute.
- Cayenne. A good food seasoning, this red pepper helps break up mucus and cholesterol. It also may improve circulation. An excellent substitute for black pepper, it is available in mild, medium, or hot varieties.
- Eggs. Purchase free-range or organic for better taste and no hormones.
- Foods for liver health. Beets, carrots, artichokes, lemons, parsnips, dandelion greens, and watercress all help keep your liver healthy.
- Millet. This tasty gluten-free whole grain is very nutritious and easy to digest.
- Nutritional yeast. Yeasts, such as brewer's, are stocked with nutrients, including B vitamins. Sprinkle these yeasts on popcorn, breads, or cereals.
- Spelt. A member of the wheat family, spelt can often be tolerated by people with gluten or wheat allergies and by people with celiac disease. It contains more protein and fiber than wheat.
- Stevia. Also known as honey leaf, stevia is a mighty herbal sweetener without the unwholesome side effects of artificial sweeteners. Just 1 to 3 drops is plenty to sweeten a cup of tea.

WOMAN TO WOMAN

She Had to Force Her Doctors to Diagnose Her

Since she was 17, Dede Wilson of Cincinnati had suffered from gastrointestinal problems that left her doctors perplexed. Specialist after specialist and years of testing failed to find the root of the problem. So Dede diagnosed herself. Her doctors scoffed at first, but they soon found out that her instinct was dead-on. Here's her story.

In the beginning, I had no clue what the problem was. I would eat lunch and then feel sick to my stomach. Nausea, vomiting, diarrhea, pain. My family doctor had no clue. He just wrote it off as nerves and prescribed Valium.

Eventually, I was referred to a gastroenterologist. Again, the tests were negative. So I received a one-size-fits-all diagnosis: irritable bowel syndrome. I endured months of useless medication.

Then, I began having irregular bleeding, which seemed odd since I was taking birth control pills to help regulate my periods. That's what pushed me over the edge. All my aunts had been telling me that I had endometriosis. They were right. In fact, it runs in our family—seven of us have it. But getting my doctors to believe it was a tremendous struggle. Every time I mentioned endometriosis, they shot it down. They said that there was no way I could have it because I was just in my early twenties. Finally, I was in so much pain I called my gynecologist and demanded treatment. He did a laparoscopy and at last diagnosed the disease correctly. I was grateful that he had found it, but I didn't feel comfortable with his treatment or bedside manner. So once again, I sought another doctor. And another. It took 4 years, but now I am seeing a physician who actually listens to my concerns.

My advice to others: Don't take a backseat to your doctor. Treating endometriosis is a partnership. If I see an article about endometriosis that I think may help my doctor understand the disease better, I mail it to him. I don't want to be just someone lying there in his office with a cloth over her naked body. I want him to know who I am and how this disease affects my life.

Peel me a grape. Bite into the fresh fruits and vegetables that you enjoy, experiment with new ones, and eat a variety of all of them, Dr. Brett urges. The phytochemicals (plant chemicals) that they contain may help ward off such catastrophic diseases as cancer, heart disease, and stroke. No one is certain how phytochemicals work, but researchers suspect that various mixtures of compounds neutralize free radicals, those unstable molecules that damage or destroy healthy cells. Since phytochemicals work as groups, you need a lot of them to make a difference. No single fruit or vegetable contains all of the phytochemicals that you need. The greater the variety of fruits and vegetables you consume, the better off you will be.

Snap up beans. Navy, pinto, lima, and other dried beans are virtually fat-free and are tremendous sources of protein that can slash or even eliminate the need for fat-laden meats in chili, stews, and salads.

To cut down on gas, soak your beans overnight in a bowl of water, then use fresh water for cooking them. Over-the-counter products such as Beano, which contains the enzyme alpha-galactosidase, also can help prevent gas by breaking down sugars in your digestive system.

Don't let meat hog your plate. Avoid letting meat crowd the fruits and vegetables off your plate. Instead, limit yourself to no more than 6 ounces of cooked meat a day. Use a small portion of meat (2 to 3 ounces after cooking) to complement, not dominate, each meal. Or, think of it this way: For every bite of meat, take four bites of fruits, vegetables, beans, and grains.

Sneak in soy. Soy contains isoflavones, which are substances that block the formation of blood vessels around new tumors, stop cancer cells from multiplying, and prevent the absorption of tumor-promoting estrogen. So instead of beef, chicken, and other meats, use soy products such as tofu, available at most grocery stores, as a main course in your meals.

Wear a milk mustache. Milk is fortified with vitamin D, which your body needs to absorb calcium. Calcium helps prevent osteoporosis, a degenerative bone disease that affects women four times more often than men. Drinking 2½ to 3 glasses of fat-free milk a day can help you reach a goal of 1,000 milligrams through your diet. Other good sources of calcium include yogurt, Cheddar cheese, sardines (with bones), tofu, and calcium-fortified orange juice.

Take your breath away. Eating one-half of an onion or a clove of garlic a day helps regulate bacteria and other organisms in both your intestines and reproductive tract. Both onion and garlic also contain a great number of cancer- and heart disease–fighting antioxidant compounds.

Heave hydrogenated foods. Foods such as commercially baked goods and margarines are often loaded with hydrogenated or partially hydrogenated oils. This means that hydrogen has been added to unsaturated fat to make it solidify. This process creates saturated fat and trans fatty acids—a gruesome pairing that raises blood levels of low-density lipoproteins (LDL), the bad cholesterol that clogs arteries. So if you read

---

THE WARNING SIGNS OF CANCER

Caught early, many cancers can be subdued. Here are the signals to look for, according to the American Cancer Society.

- Any change in bowel or bladder habits
- A sore that does not heal
- A lump or thickening in the breast or elsewhere
- Unusual bleeding or discharge
- Chronic indigestion or swallowing problems
- An obvious change in a wart or a mole
- A nagging cough or hoarseness

In most cases, these signs are symptoms of some disease other than cancer. But to be on the safe side, if you notice any of them, notify your doctor immediately. If it does turn out that you have cancer, the sooner you get started on treatment, the better your chances will be for a complete recovery and a long, healthy life.

---

the word *hydrogenated* on a food label, put the package back on the grocery shelf.

Reach for a supplement. Getting adequate amounts of all the nutrients that you need to stay healthy can be a challenge, even if you eat a well-balanced diet, so take a once-a-day multivitamin. It should include 100 percent of the Daily Values for calcium, magnesium, niacin, iron, folic acid, chromium, and vitamins A, C, D, E, and B_{12}. In particular, the antioxidant vitamins in these preparations will help prevent heart disease and other tissue damage.

Jump-Start Your Exercise Routine

Regular exercise has long been known to reduce the risk of heart disease and stroke among women, but that's not all.

(continued on page 22)

YOUR TREE OF KNOWLEDGE

Research your family history of ailments by talking to your parents, grandparents, aunts, uncles, and siblings. If a blood relative has a disease or condition, you need not panic, but you should be aware that you are at an increased risk.

The more relatives you talk to, the better. You should also know something about their lifestyles. For example, did they drink or smoke?

Serious but potentially preventable conditions are the ones you should pay the most attention to, including cancer, high blood pressure, diabetes, alcoholism, heart disease, and depression.

The sample family tree below depicts ways that you can chart your family's medical history. (Deceased members are crossed out, with ages of death in circles next to them.)

Sample Family Tree

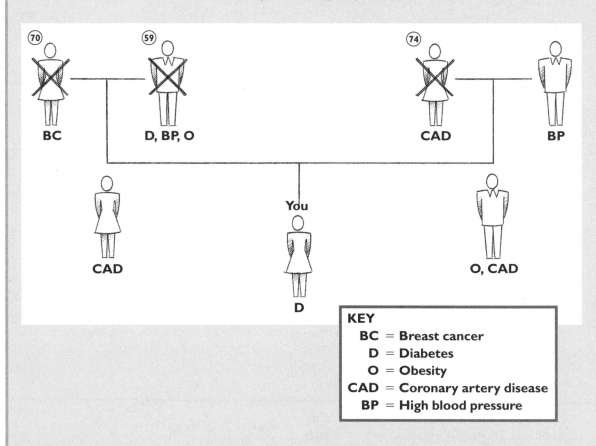

KEY

BC = Breast cancer
D = Diabetes
O = Obesity
CAD = Coronary artery disease
BP = High blood pressure

Organize your findings into a chart as shown in the sample. This will allow you to view the medical histories of several of your relatives all at once. You'll need to assign a letter to each medical condition or disease that occurs in your family and place that letter under each affected relative. Use the key to note which conditions the letters represent. Also note the age of death if the relative is deceased.

When your medical family tree is as complete as you can make it, review it with your physician to get a clearer understanding of your risks.

Your Family Tree

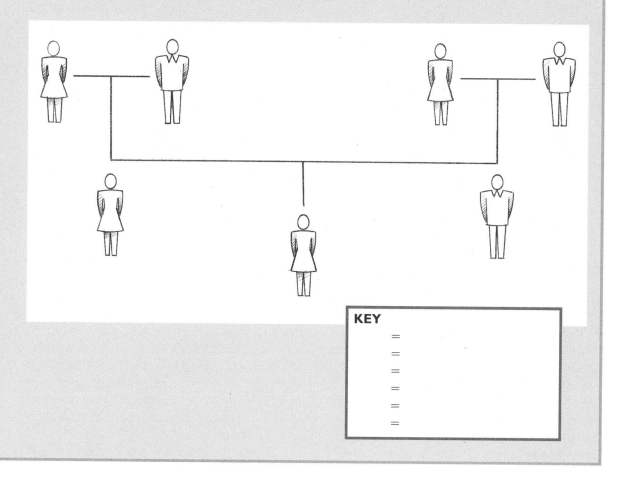

KEY

=

=

=

=

=

=

Women who exercise an hour a day may also reduce their risk of breast cancer by 20 percent, according to findings from the Nurses' Health Study, one of the largest studies (involving 121,701 women) ever done on women's health. Other researchers who have evaluated data from the Nurses' Health Study found that women who did the most weekly exercise had significantly lower risks of developing type 2 diabetes than did women who exercised the least.

Weight-bearing exercise, such as walking, jogging, and running, can also help women maintain bone mass and derail osteoporosis—the thinning and wearing away of bone that occurs as we get older, says Marianne Legato, M.D., founder and director of the Partnership for Women's Health at Columbia University College of Physicians and Surgeons in New York City and author of *What Women Need to Know*.

Simply walking 40 minutes a day, four times a week, can make an enormous difference in your body's ability to defend itself against a multitude of ailments.

Rest Easy

Sleep helps your body rebuild muscle tissue and replenish chemicals in your brain. Without adequate sleep—typically, 7 to 9 hours a night— you may be less energetic and more irritable, have greater difficulty concentrating, and be more prone to accidents, Dr. Brett says. Taking 200 to 300 milligrams of calcium and of magnesium every evening can help you get more restful sleep, she adds.

Valerian, an herbal remedy, has been shown to

HOW TO BE A HEALTH DETECTIVE

Resources abound, both in bookstores and on the Internet, for getting information about your health or a particular illness that may be challenging you. Here a few book titles you can find at the public library.

- *Mayo Clinic Family Health Book* and *The American Medical Association Family Medical Guide*, used together, provide basic health information in easy-to-understand language. *Mayo Clinic Family Health Book* provides information on more than 1,000 ailments and disorders. *The American Medical Association Family Medical Guide* includes illustrations and diagnoses for common symptoms.

- *Health Care Almanac: Every Person's Guide to the Thoughtful and Practical Sides of Medicine*, by the American Medical Association, is arranged in alphabetical order with addresses of medical associations and a variety of health-related information.

- *The Female Body: An Owner's Manual*, by the editors of *Prevention* Magazine Health Books, is designed to answer many concerns that women have about their health.

- *Our Bodies, Ourselves for the New Century*, by the Boston Women's Health Book Collective staff, continues to be considered the best in providing women with comprehensive coverage of health care.

---

have tranquilizing and sedative properties similar to the prescription drug diazepam (Valium), but without the side effects. Plus, valerian is nonaddictive. Dr. Brett suggests taking two 400-milligram capsules 30 minutes before bedtime. Valerian is also sold as a tea, but Dr. Brett says that it stinks like dirty, old socks and can be difficult to drink. Do not use valerian with sleep-enhancing or mood-regulating medications, because it may intensify their effects. It may cause heart palpitations and nervousness in sensitive individuals. If it stimulates you that way, discontinue using it. Valerian is available at most health food stores.

In addition, according to Dr. Brett, heeding

For information that's constantly brought up-to-date, both medical and public libraries are equipped with collections of electronic databases and Internet connections. Here are some Internet sites to look for.

- Healthfinder (www.healthfinder.gov), a government Web site, offers a searchable topic interface with additional links to professional organizations, academic institutions, and libraries.

- The American College of Obstetricians and Gynecologists Web site (www.acog.org) addresses a variety of women's health issues.

- CancerNet (http://cancernet.nci.nih.gov) from the National Cancer Institute provides current cancer information covering diagnosis, treatment, and cancer physicians and facilities.

- The National Women's Health Information Center (www.4woman.org) is maintained by the U.S. Department of Health and Human Services. Updated health-related news stories, consumer information, and links to medical dictionaries and glossaries are features of this Web site.

- The North American Menopause Society Web site (www.menopause.org) discusses scientific studies related to menopause.

the following advice also can help you sleep better.

Stick to a schedule. Try to go to bed and wake up at approximately the same times each day.

Kick back and unwind. Take a few moments before you turn in for the night to unload the stresses of the day through meditation or deep breathing. And avoid doing strenuous exercise an hour or two before you go to bed. The physical and psychological stimulation may wire you up.

Drink milk or herbal tea. Milk is loaded with L-tryptophan, which helps some people sleep. Drinking a cup of herbal tea before bed is a soothing ritual that can help you relax.

Avoid alcohol and caffeine. Either one of these substances, taken up to 8 hours before bed, will disrupt your natural sleep patterns.

Eat light. A large dinner or late-night snack might keep you tossing and turning as your digestive tract works overtime.

Strangle Stress

Women, particularly mothers, are more likely than men to feel stressed, according to a survey by Roper Starch Worldwide, a marketing research and consulting firm based in New York City.

While 21 percent of women in 30 countries report feeling an immense amount of stress, only 15 percent of men share those feelings. Among the most stressed women in the world are full-time working mothers with children under the age of 13, with nearly one in four feeling stress almost every day. More single women than single men around the world feel intense daily stress, and the number of stressed separated or divorced women exceeds that of stressed separated or divorced men by a 3-to-2 margin.

Of course, excessive stress is more than just a nuisance. It can make women more susceptible to infections and hormonal imbalances, Dr. Brett says. Meditation, yoga, and other techniques can go a long way toward reducing the stress that you feel and, in turn, reduce your risk of disease.

Listening to music is the number one stress-buster for more than half of the world's women, according to Roper Starch Worldwide. Reading,

WOMEN ASK WHY

How do I get a mammogram if I'm a AA-cup kinda woman?

Although smaller-breasted women may be concerned about whether an adequate mammogram can be done on them, they should be assured that the size of their breasts doesn't matter, even if they are A or AA cups. Technicians seldom have to treat small-breasted women differently from women who have larger breasts. The compression is the same. It doesn't hurt any more or less if you have smaller breasts.

But the truly important message here is for small-breasted women to get annual mammograms after age 40 like everyone else. Some women with smaller breasts may think that they are at lower risk for cancer because they have less breast tissue. But that's not true. Breast cancer is no more common among large-breasted women than among smaller-breasted women. No matter how much breast tissue she has, every woman has the same percentage of risk as any other woman in her age group.

Expert consulted
Deborah Capko, M.D.
Breast surgeon and associate medical director
Institute for Breast Care at Hackensack
University Medical Center
New Jersey

walking, or taking a bath or shower are other popular ways to unwind.

Make an Annual Pilgrimage

Regular physical exams and medical tests can help detect small problems in your body before they get big. The type and number of tests you'll need each year will depend on many factors, including your age and previous medical history. But here are a few critical tests that women older than 40 should undergo, according to Dr. Legato. Some of them may be familiar and a regular part of life. Others may not be, and in those cases, you should ask your doctor about adding them to your schedule of routine medical care.

- A blood pressure reading by a doctor or nurse at least once a year. High blood pressure (readings consistently above 140/90) is a risk factor for stroke and heart disease.
- A mammogram at least every other year after age 40 can help detect breast cancer.
- A manual breast exam by a knowledgeable physician once a year, in addition to a mammogram.
- A complete head-to-toe skin exam by a knowledgeable physician once a year.
- A cholesterol screening once a year. Since heart disease is the number one killer of women, Dr. Legato believes that monitoring total cholesterol, LDL, high-density lipoproteins (HDL), and triglycerides is an essential component of preventive care.
- A thyroid-function test every year after age 50. For this test, your blood sample is analyzed at a laboratory.
- A bone-density screening to help determine your risk of developing osteoporosis. You only have to have this test done once.
- A serum estradiol test every 2 years after age 45. Low blood levels of estradiol (less than 50 picograms/deciliter) may mean that you need hormone-replacement therapy.

- An electrocardiogram (EKG) every year. More than one in three heart attacks that occur in women are silent, without any outward warning signals. An EKG can help determine if you've had any heart damage in the previous year.
- A fecal occult blood test every year after age 50. This test can disclose any hidden blood in your stool that may be a warning sign of colon cancer and other diseases.
- A digital rectal exam once a year. In this test, which Dr. Legato highly recommends, a physician inserts a gloved finger into your rectum and feels for growths, abnormalities, and signs of bleeding.

"I use it all of the time," Dr. Legato says, "and I think many more women's lives would be saved, in terms of death from colon cancer, by an early detection of polyps in the colon. It can take years for those polyps to become cancerous, but all become malignant eventually. Some of the cardinal ways to detect them are with a simple digital examination and by testing the stool for blood."

In between these tests, always be sure to do monthly skin and breast self-examinations at home, Dr. Ferry urges.

Manage Your Meds

Medicines can heal, but they also can harm. In fact, in ancient Greece, *pharmakos*, the root word of pharmacy, meant both remedy and poison. So be careful whenever you take medicines. In particular, be wary of drug interactions.

Dr. Ferry urges that your primary-care physician should know all of the medications, both prescription and over-the-counter, that you're taking. And don't forget about herbal remedies and other alternative treatments that you may be ingesting. Like any drugs, these remedies can cause side effects or interact with other drugs. Some herbs, such as chaparral, can trigger hepatitis and other liver damage. Before you leave your doctor's office, pharmacy, or alternative health-care provider's office with a new drug, make certain that you fully understand how to take the drug properly. Be sure to ask the following questions.

- What is the name of the drug and what will it do?
- How often should I take it?
- When should I take it?
- If I forget to take it, what should I do?
- What side effects might I expect, and should I report them?
- Will I need periodic blood or urine tests to monitor adverse effects?
- Is there any information about this drug that I can take home with me?

In addition, keep in an easy-to-find place in your purse or wallet a list of all medications that you are taking—again, including over-the-counter drugs and complementary treatments—and their dosages, Dr. Ferry says. That could be extremely helpful in an emergency, if you're incapacitated and can't communicate with the health-care professionals trying to save your life.

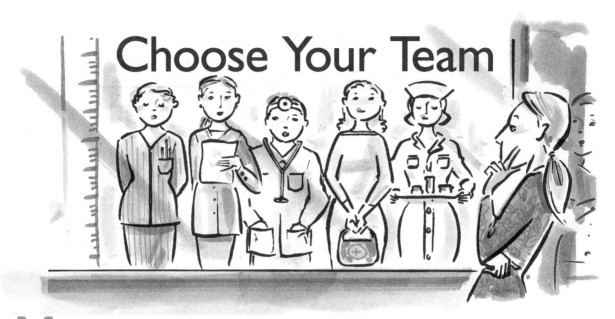

Choose Your Team

Many of us spend more time and effort on locating a good hairdresser than on finding a good doctor. Who can blame us? Shopping for doctors is intimidating. They all hang diplomas—written in Latin, which no one understands—on every wall of their offices, so we presume they're extremely well-educated. And most are not exactly fond of being interviewed about their competency by people who know nothing about medicine. But finding the right doctor is something we all need to do—and we need to do it now, when we're well, not when we're on the way to the hospital.

To complicate matters even more, as women, we have special health issues that our doctors should be familiar with. Can your doctor, for instance, give female-specific advice about preventing heart disease? Can she answer your questions about hormone-replacement therapy? Does she know enough about alternative medicine—herbs, supplements, and the like—to have an intelligent conversation with you about any alternative treatments you are using? Maybe you have both a regular and an alternative doctor. Wouldn't it be wonderful if the two of them could talk together about your care once in a while? Wouldn't it be nice if your health-care team were as good a match for you as your hairdresser is? Here's how to make that happen.

Finding Dr. Right

Nowadays, two types of doctors perform the role formerly played by the general practitioner: the family practitioner and the internist. While doctors in both of these specialties receive similar training, there are some significant differences between them.

Family practitioners study general adult medicine as well as pediatrics, gynecology, obstetrics, and in-office surgical procedures. So their training is broad. Internists, on the other hand, receive more in-depth training in the diagnosis and treatment of adult illnesses, such as diabetes and heart disease.

Gynecologists also sometimes act as primary-care doctors for women. They can offer some preventive care, monitor your blood pressure and cholesterol, and do screening tests for thyroid function and colon cancer. But gynecology is actually a medical-surgical specialty, and a gynecologist's skills are best used to treat illness of your reproductive organs.

One of the best ways to find a competent doctor is to ask around, but don't ask just anyone. If you can, question people who work in the medical field. Emergency room physicians and nurses are often in a good position to judge the abilities of local doctors. If it's a gynecologist you're after, ask midwives and nurse practitioners, says Karla Morales, vice president of communications for People's Medical Society, a non-profit organization devoted to consumer health issues, in Allentown, Pennsylvania.

Doctor-referral services can also be somewhat helpful, but you need to be aware of their limitations. Listed in the yellow pages, these services are usually run either by a local hospital, which lists only doctors employed there, or by a county medical society, which is a paid-membership organization.

At the least-sophisticated level, these services simply give callers the names of doctors from a rotating list of members. The better services, on the other hand, list basic information concerning board-certification and specialties of their doctors. And most of them weed out doctors who are trouble or who have been the subject of numerous complaints. "But these services do not give true comparisons or negative information about doctors," says Morales. For that information, contact the American Board of Medical Specialties at 1007 Church Street, Suite 404, Evanston, Illinois 60201.

WOMEN ASK WHY

Is it better for me to see a doctor who's a woman rather than one who's a man?

It's true that female doctors are more likely than male doctors to offer advice on preventing illness. They also tend to be better listeners and are less likely to interrupt their patients. But, on average, they rate only slightly better—10 percent—at these skills than male doctors. In fact, differences among female doctors are often greater than the average difference between male and female doctors.

So making female gender your number one priority when you're doctor shopping isn't necessarily going to find you the best doctor in your area. It's probably better to look for a doctor, male or female, who encourages you to ask questions, listens to you, explains things clearly, and treats you with respect.

However, when it comes to intimate personal examinations, women and men tend to be more comfortable and more frank with someone of their own gender and ethnicity. A woman who is uncomfortable with a pelvic or breast examination usually prefers seeing a female gynecologist for her care. Maybe that's one reason that female doctors now make up the majority of gynecologists.

Expert consulted
Erica Frank, M.D.
Associate professor in the department of
    family and preventive medicine
Emory University School of Medicine
Atlanta

Taking the Alternate Route

If you're looking for a doctor practicing alternative medicine, consider a naturopathic doctor, or N.D. An N.D. is trained in all forms of alternative medicine, including nutrition and herbal remedies. Look for one who is a member of the American Association of Naturopathic Physicians (AANP). These doctors have all graduated from one of the four U.S. or Canadian colleges recognized by the Council on Naturopathic Medical Education.

To find an N.D. in your area, you can check the AANP's Web site at www.naturopathic.org. Or for a small fee, you can receive a national membership list and a brochure describing naturopathic physicians and their services from the AANP, 601 Valley Street, Suite 105, Seattle, WA 98109-4229.

Eleven states license N.D.'s., and four states (Connecticut, Montana, Washington, and Alaska) require that health insurance providers cover N.D. care. In states where N.D.'s are not licensed, anyone can claim to be a naturopathic doctor, so checking credentials and education is important.

What about Dentists?

If you're looking for a dentist, experts again suggest that you ask for help from people you know and trust, including health-care professionals such as your doctor. You can also call to ask faculty members of the nearest dental school, which is often associated with a medical school. About three out of four dentists also belong to the American Dental Association (ADA), which means that they have some interest in continuing education and maintaining a professional practice, says Kimberly Harms, D.D.S., a dentist from Farmington, Minnesota, and consumer advisor for the ADA. The ADA can give you a list of its members in your area. Contact them at the ADA, 211 East Chicago Avenue, Chicago, IL 60611. You can also request information via e-mail on their Web site at www.ada.org.

The staff of the dentist's office should allow you to come in to look around or to have a get-acquainted visit with the dentist, where you

> ### WHAT TO LOOK FOR IN A FIRST-RATE HOSPITAL
>
> Generally, your doctor, not you, chooses the hospital you will go into for surgery. So if you want to go to a particular hospital, you'll have to become the patient of a doctor who has operating or attending privileges there. Good doctors are more likely to be affiliated with good hospitals, but how can you be certain that your doctor is sending you to the best hospital for *your* problem? According to Karla Morales, vice president of communications for People's Medical Society, here are some things to consider.
>
> ❥ Is the hospital accredited? About 80 percent of U.S. hospitals are accredited by either the Joint Commission on Accreditation of Healthcare Organizations or the American Osteopathic Association. This means the facility is inspected every 3 years for a long list of items.
>
> ❥ Is the staff top-quality? The doctors who will be treating you in the hospital should be board-certified by their specialties' professional societies. Find out, too, how the hospital is equipped to treat your particular illness or to perform your type of surgery. How often do they treat your kind of illness? What success rates do they have? You can start with a phone call to the hospital administration office for answers to these questions. Studies show that hospitals get better at procedures they often perform, and the results are better, too.

simply discuss your concerns and get to know each other, Dr. Harms says. A good dentist will have a clean, organized office and friendly staff; will use proper sterilization techniques, including wearing a face mask and gloves; will take a comprehensive dental and medical history before working on you; and will openly discuss treatment options and fees, she says. Many dentists these days work with a dental hygienist, who cleans your teeth, so you'll want to meet the dental hygienist as well.

By the way, D.D.S. and D.M.D. degrees are basically the same thing.

- Is there an all-R.N. staff? The best hospitals have moved in this direction, replacing practical nurses and others with more highly trained R.N.'s.

- What's the staffing level? Make sure that the hospital is not understaffed. One nurse for every three to eight patients can help assure good care. You can obtain information about a hospital's nursing staff from the hospital itself, your state affiliate to the American Nurses Association, or the American Hospital Association.

- What is the hospital's infection rate? The national average for infections acquired in hospitals is growing, but most infections are avoidable. In fact, the Harvard Medical Practice Study in 1991 found that 70 percent of all wound infections could be prevented when proper procedures are followed.

- What are the hospital's morbidity (nonfatal complications) and mortality statistics for your procedure? While this does not tell you everything, it gives you a measure for comparison of one hospital with another.

Get information from your doctor and local hospitals, but also ask other health-care professionals, clergy, and business leaders. If there is a major quality difference among hospitals, your sources are likely to tell you. If there is a doctor in your region who is well-regarded for her work, find out at which hospital she works.

All about Counselors and Therapists

As anyone who has ever tangled with depression will tell you, emotional well-being plays an important role in overall good health—but finding the right therapist can be tricky. If you've never used one before, you may not even know what to look for.

The following guidelines can help you identify a therapist who is both professionally qualified and the best personal match for you.

You should feel comfortable. You need to trust this person enough to openly talk about your thoughts, feelings, and behavior, says Faith Tanney, Ph.D., a psychologist practicing in Washington, D.C. "You may feel challenged or disagree with things, but you should have a basic trust in the therapist and feel as though she is listening and interested in you and understands who you are."

It may take about two sessions to decide if you feel comfortable working with a particular therapist, Dr. Tanney says.

The therapist should act like a professional. Psychologists and other mental health professionals are expected to adhere to a code of ethics that includes confidentiality and certain boundaries. Those boundaries involve not having an outside relationship with a client while she's in treatment; not counseling someone with whom there is a preexisting relationship, such as friend, employee, or student; not having any kind of sexual contact with the client; and structuring financial arrangements clearly and honestly.

Warning signs of a lack of professionalism manifest themselves when the therapist is often late beginning or ending sessions, takes phone calls during sessions, confuses you with other clients, forgets what you've said in past sessions, or talks about herself instead of keeping the primary focus on you, advises Dr. Tanney.

The therapist should work with you to establish treatment goals. In these days of managed care, you're lucky if your insurance company pays for six treatment sessions. Focusing on your central issues and setting goals to help resolve those issues is the best use of your

WOMEN ASK WHY

Why do people sometimes go into the hospital well and come out sick?

Hospitals are full of sick people, and sick people are sometimes contagious. Organisms can be transmitted in the air, by direct human contact, on towels and sheets, via the housekeeping crew, by contact with surgical wounds, and through the use of urinary catheters, drainage tubes, and ventilator tubes. Studies show that most people don't develop a hospital-acquired infection until at least 72 hours after admission, so some infections may not become apparent until after you've been discharged from the hospital.

How can you protect yourself? Ask your doctor about the hospital's track record for infections. (People at the hospital itself may paint too rosy a picture.) Make sure all hospital personnel who come in contact with you wash their hands. Ask them to do so in your room, in your presence.

Nurses who wear fake fingernails are more likely to harbor harmful organisms than those who don't. In a recent study, 68 percent of nurses wearing fake nails were carrying harmful bacteria on their hands even after washing, so ask nurses who wear fake nails to put on gloves before treating you.

If you're concerned that a sick roommate has something you could catch, ask your doctor or nurse about your risk. Change your room at once if there is any chance that you could become infected.

If you're undergoing a procedure that requires the removal of hair, refuse to be shaven the night before surgery. A low rate of infection is achieved by using a chemical depilatory or barber clippers to remove hair on the morning of the surgery.

If you have a urinary catheter, a nurse should check it regularly to make sure that it is draining correctly. This may help you avoid a urinary tract infection.

Expert consulted
Karla Morales
Vice president of communications
People's Medical Society

time, Dr. Tanney says. For this, a therapist needs to be focused.

The therapist should empower you. A good therapist doesn't attempt to solve problems for you. At best, she provides helpful insights and offers new ways of looking at your situation, serving more as a catalyst to help you develop the ability to problem solve for yourself, Dr. Tanney says.

The therapist should have good credentials. Many different types of professionals, including the following, practice psychotherapy. Psychiatrists are, essentially, physicians, and with a few exceptions, they are the only mental health professionals licensed to prescribe drugs. Clinical or counseling psychologists (Ph.D., Psy.D., or Ed.D.) spend an average of 7 years in postgraduate school developing expertise in human behavior, diagnosis, and treatment. Clinical social workers (M.S.W.) have earned master's degrees in social work and are trained in individual, family, and group counseling with an emphasis on tapping community resources. Psychiatric advanced nurse practitioners (R.N.) are registered nurses with advanced training in the prevention and treatment of mental health problems. And marriage and family therapists have earned, at minimum, master's degrees and are specialists in their respective fields.

Licensure is an important credential. Through licensure you can be certain that an independent review of the professional's training and experience has been conducted. All physicians, psychologists, nurses, and social workers are licensed in every state. Marriage and family therapists are licensed in most states. Most insurance companies require licensure for payment for mental health services, and licensure also assures that you'll have legal recourse if inappropriate care is provided.

When Should You Fire Your Doctor?

What if you're seeing a doctor you just don't care for? No doctor is perfect—you have to balance her strengths and weaknesses. You may want to discuss your dissatisfactions with her before you start shopping for a new doctor. There may be room for reconciliation.

Still, most experts say that it's time to end the relationship if your doctor puts you down or judges you, fails to exercise good medical judgment, orders the same test several times when once would do, does not perform thorough physical exams, or minimizes serious side effects or risks of a treatment. Likewise, think about going elsewhere if your doctor blocks your attempts at communication or makes you feel so intimidated that you don't speak up, isn't interested in your worries and concerns, ignores psychological and social causes of illness as well as job-related health problems, or is disrespectful or verbally abusive to you or others.

DOES YOUR DOCTOR HAVE THE RIGHT STUFF?

Whether the doctor you're considering is traditional or alternative, you need to check her credentials and other more subjective aspects of her practice, says Karla Morales, vice president of communications for People's Medical Society. Call the doctor's office for this information. It's a good way to find out if her staff is consumer-friendly and willing to answer your questions. Here are some of the questions you should ask.

- Is the doctor accepting new patients?
- Is the doctor board-certified? Board certification means that the doctor has taken extra training and passed the vigorous examination given by a national board of professionals in that specialty field. Board certification is an important way by which doctors judge their colleagues' credentials. Keep in mind that alternative physicians are not likely to be board-certified.
- Does the doctor have get-acquainted visits? How long are they? (Expect 10 to 15 minutes.) How much do they cost?
- At what hospitals does the doctor have privileges to admit, treat, or operate on her patients? Privileges are rights granted to a doctor by a hospital review board, depending on the hospital's need for doctors and on a doctor's qualifications.
- Does the doctor accept phone calls from patients? At what hours? Does she have e-mail? The doctor's staff can frequently answer questions over the phone, but you should have access to the doctor herself if you feel that's necessary.
- Does she have any evening or weekend hours?
- How far in advance is the doctor booked for routine appointments? How quickly can you get in for an emergency?
- Does the doctor work in a group? How many doctors are in the group? Are they all board-certified? Who backs up the doctor when she's on vacation?
- Does she work in conjunction with alternative practitioners or make referrals to them?

Time Is Health

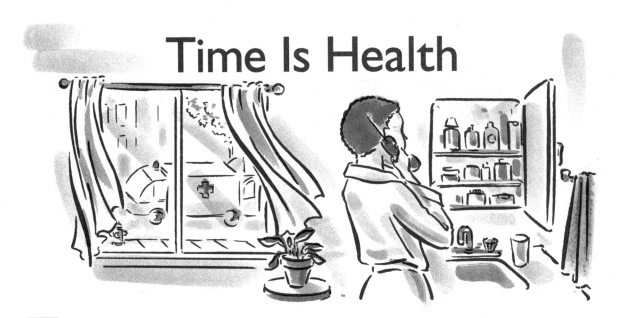

To call or not to call? That is the question.

We've all asked it, maybe during a moment of breathlessness . . . or in the middle of a high fever . . . or after the onset of an odd chill and insistent pain in one arm. Sometimes, illness strikes suddenly and without warning.

Should we dial 911, maybe head for the nearest hospital emergency room? If we do decide we need to get to an ER, how can we be sure we'll get the best care available? The best doctors? The best medications?

The time to consider these questions is *not* when you're anxious—maybe even panicked—over your health. The time to think about them is now.

Take Some Urgency Out of Emergencies

Selecting an emergency-care site ahead of time is barely more appealing than buying your own cemetery plot, but it's a lot more important. The choice of hospital could be lifesaving for heart attack victims, according to one major study published in the *New England Journal of Medicine*. People treated at hospitals where high volumes of heart attack patients are seen were more likely to survive than those who went to "low-volume" hospitals.

So plan your emergency options before you need them. Here's how.

Start with your doctor. Ask your physician where she practices. Then, ask what specialized care the hospital offers, says Barbara N. Wynn, M.D., an attending physician in the emergency department at Spectrum Health Downtown Hospital in Grand Rapids, Michigan.

Be sure about insurance. Avoid paperwork nightmares by identifying which area facilities your health insurance will accept, says Julie A. Johnson, Pharm.D., associate professor of pharmacy practice at the University of Florida College of Pharmacy in Gainesville.

Check the ratings. Hospitals are graded by national groups such as the Joint Commission on Accreditation of Healthcare Organizations (JCAHO). To find a facility's rating, call the hospital to ask, or search the Internet for JCAHO's Web site, which provides ratings information.

Map out your move. You could get to the video store blindfolded—how about to the ER? In heavy fog? With a broken wrist? Rehearse the route so you don't have to worry about getting lost or delayed when time counts, suggests Laura Bontempo, M.D., an attending emergency physician in the department of emergency medicine at Brigham and Women's Hospital in Boston.

Give your name, rank, and allergies. On a small piece of heavy paper, write your name, address, allergies, chronic conditions, physician's name and number, health insurance account number, medications, and emergency contact person. Put it in your wallet next to your driver's license, says Dr. Bontempo. It will speak for you if you can't.

Care for your kids. An ER visit is hard on children who accompany a parent in distress. Arrange a backup adult who can look after little ones, urges Dr. Bontempo, and put that person's name and number in your wallet.

Fill your peace-of-mind prescription. Where's your nearest 24-hour pharmacy? This is a trick question if it's 2:00 A.M. and you're out of pain medicine. Next to the phone, post the number and location of your nearest relief *now*. Ditto, your community's poison control center number.

IS YOUR MEDICATION TOO "MANLY"?

In or out of the emergency room, it's likely that the drugs you are given were scantily tested on women. "Except for drugs involving sex hormones, we have a vast number of drugs that have very limited studies in safety and effectiveness for women," says Julie A. Johnson, Pharm.D., associate professor of pharmacy practice at the University of Florida College of Pharmacy in Gainesville.

This imbalance is no secret. Before 1993, drug companies routinely excluded premenopausal women from many trials to guard against possible injury to fetuses. As mounting research demonstrated that drugs proven to work on men weren't necessarily effective on women, the FDA, which regulates prescription and nonprescription medications in the United States, realized that it needed to change its gender prescription. In 1993, it revised its guidelines to promote more participation by women in clinical drug trials.

In the years since, not much has happened. Pregnant and lactating women are barred from drug tests, and pretrial pregnancy screening is a given. Research on gender differences and drugs is still far from definitive. As a paper in an international pharmacology journal concedes, "Little is known about drug effects in women when compared to men."

The issue isn't about differences in body size, explains Dr. Johnson, but in how we use, absorb, and process drugs. "I could give an 80-milligram dose of something to both a 100-pound woman and a 200-pound man, and the man could actually have a higher concentration of the drug in his blood."

While research in medication use and gender is at a very early stage, Dr. Johnson believes that safety isn't a concern. "Most of the drugs we use are so safe that any differences don't cause problems." To help even the balance in knowledge about how drugs affect women, she offers these hints.

Take part in testing. When you see a newspaper ad recruiting women for a clinical drug trial, grab the chance.

Ask, listen, talk. When a medication is prescribed, ask questions: What is it for? What are potential side effects? And let your medical professional know how you're feeling once you start your medication.

Get Help Now!

If you're unsure whether your symptoms are telling you to get to an ER or to just make an appointment with your doctor, you have lots of company. Of more than 90 million ER visits in the United States each year, only about half can be called urgent. Some mishaps, of course, are easy calls: losing an argument with the garbage disposal and spurting blood all over the sink, for example, or seeing a bone poking up after a fall. But some less obvious symptoms, while not always screaming, "Emergency!" can be vital cues to call 911.

Dr. Bontempo listens to patient concerns in the emergency room all day. There are two in particular that push her heart rate up: "When patients say, 'I feel like someone's standing on my chest' and 'I have the worst headache I've ever had.'" According to Dr. Bontempo, these symptoms say that it's probably time to get to the ER.

Chest discomfort. Is it indigestion—or a heart attack? Since it's tough for even the best medics to differentiate, says Dr. Bontempo, "chest pain is a complaint that we take very seriously." You should, too. Heart disease is the leading cause of death for American women.

Other signs of a heart attack include difficulty breathing; sweating; nausea; weakness; radiation of pain to your arms, especially your left arm, or to your jaw; and a sense of impending doom, she says.

"Worst headache of your life." If it's your all-time skull-splitter, it could be one of several serious problems, including bleeding in your brain, Dr. Bontempo advises. Extreme headache

WOMAN TO WOMAN
Speaking Up Saved Her Life . . . Twice

Heart and blood problems make medical issues extra complicated for Ellen Levine, but her mouth works perfectly. That's why this Internet search editor, of East Setauket, New York, is alive today at age 53. Here's her story.

I have a fairly common heart condition called mitral valve prolapse. It can cause crushing chest pressure that feels like a heart attack.

Last year, I started having chest pain that got progressively worse over several weeks. My cardiologist decided to give me a cardiac catheter test, in which a small tube is inserted into the heart to check for abnormalities—usually a simple procedure. But not in my case.

I have two blood problems: one is a condition that makes me bleed for too long, and the other is an antibody that can produce clots in my blood vessels. So before the cardiologist could do the test, I needed to take both a blood thinner and a special clotting enhancer. The morning I was scheduled for the catheter, I met with my blood specialist. He stressed that I had to have the clotting enhancer at least 1 hour before the procedure, or else I could bleed uncontrollably.

So when my nurse told me that it was time to transfer me from one hospital to another for the catheter, I told her I couldn't go. "You have to give me the clotting enhancer first," I told her.

can also indicate infection, especially if it is coupled with a fever, she says.

Stomach or abdominal pain. Maybe it was the ham sandwich . . . but it could also be an ectopic, or tubal, pregnancy. More potential villains and the locations of their pain are a perforated stomach ulcer (upper abdomen), gallstones (right upper abdomen), and appendicitis (around your navel, to the lower right side). Sudden, severe pain in general is a red flag.

I knew from talking to the blood specialist that my medicines were delivered intravenously, through separate IVs, and I had been given only the blood thinner. The nurse checked the book, and sure enough, I was right.

She was thrilled. "You don't know how many people don't know their own medications," she told me.

Just after she started the IV for the second medication, the transport people came to move me, and once again I had to take control of the situation.

"I can come with you in 27 minutes," I said to them. "Go have a cup of coffee."

The procedure went like clockwork, and the results were 100 percent clean.

If I hadn't spoken up, there is every chance I'd have bled to death. Keeping quiet could have killed me—and this wasn't the first time.

As an Internet search editor working with press queries every day, I got lots of questions about year 2000 (Y2K) compliance. That got me thinking about my own cardiac defibrillator implant, a specially programmed device that helps regulate my heart rate with electrical current. So during a regular checkup on the defibrillator, I jokingly asked the nurse, "By the way, this is Y2K compliant, isn't it?" She laughed, checked with the manufacturer, and reported back: No, it wasn't. So it had to be reprogrammed. Otherwise, I might not have been around to greet the new millennium.

Loss of consciousness. No ifs, ands, or buts—call an ambulance or get someone to take you to the ER now.

Trouble breathing. Do you have asthma? Then you're almost twice as likely as a man to end up in the ER with a severe attack, according to research. A cramped air supply could also signal emphysema, heart failure, or a blood clot in your lung. If you suspect an allergic reaction to an insect bite, food, or medication, call for an ambulance immediately, advises Dr. Bontempo.

Allergic reactions can progress fast, and trained paramedics can make a major difference in the outcome.

Poisoning. Check the product label for instructions, and call your community poison control center. If an ER visit is necessary, take the product with you in its original container, says Dr. Bontempo. If you're not sure which product was consumed, take any medications or potentially poisonous items that could be the culprit, she adds.

Sudden blindness. If sight fails suddenly in one or both eyes—even for an instant—hit the phone. It could be a stroke; without care, that sight loss could be permanent.

Unexplained stupor or disorientation. The reasons could range from low blood sugar to drug overdose to stroke. Whatever the cause, "you need to find out," says Dr. Bontempo.

Coughing or vomiting blood. If a small quantity of blood comes up, call your primary physician, says Dr. Bontempo. But if you're bringing up much more than a tablespoon of blood and your instincts say that something serious is happening, the ER is where you should be.

Cold arm or leg pain. A moment ago, your arm was fine; now it feels cold. You may have a blood clot in an artery, says Dr. Bontempo. If circulation is cut off for more than 6 hours, the extremity could be damaged permanently, so get to the ER as soon as possible.

Swollen arm or leg. If one of your extremities, especially your calf, is swollen, you could have a blood clot in a deep vein, warns Dr. Bontempo. If the clot migrates to your lungs, it could clog your bloodflow, so get some emergency medical attention. Female smokers who take birth control pills are at a higher risk for blood clots, she adds.

Severe or continued vomiting. "This can lead to severe dehydration: definitely an emergency situation regardless of the cause," says Dr. Bontempo.

Suicidal feelings. Does the person's state pose a danger to herself or others? Get her to the ER, urges Dr. Bontempo, so psychological help can be consulted.

Vaginal bleeding. When it occurs in an otherwise healthy, pregnant woman in the second or third trimester, quick attention is important, says Dr. Bontempo. It could be a signal that the baby is in distress. If you are not pregnant and you're bleeding through more than one pad an hour during an otherwise normal period, a trip to the ER is in order.

Worst Come, First Served

A siren wails, lights flash, and the next thing you know, emergency medical technicians are wheeling you into the ER.

And then what? Filling out insurance forms while you bleed all over a gurney? That's a nightmare many of us share, but the law says that you needn't worry. You're more important than paperwork. Federal legislation requires that "every patient who presents to the emergency room has to have a screening exam and be stabilized," regardless of insurance, assures one expert.

ERs are not in business to perform "wallet biopsies," says Dr. Wynn. "Our first priority is to take care of patients."

REAL-LIFE SCENARIO
She Found a Lump in Her Breast and Is Watching It

Abbie, 47, has never been one to panic over anything. So recently, when she felt something small and hard, like a grain of uncooked rice, in her left breast while taking a shower, she didn't think much of it. She was accustomed to giving herself a monthly breast exam, so she figured she'd just keep an eye on it. If it was anything serious, she would feel it growing and go to her doctor. After all, there was no history of breast cancer in her family, and a mammogram 18 months before had been perfectly clear, so there was little likelihood of her having any real problem. When she mentioned her discovery to her sister, Julia, however, she found herself in hot water. It was all she could do to keep Julia from dragging her to the hospital immediately. What should she do to calm her sister's fears: talk her out of her panic or give in and waste a lot of money on a "useless" doctor's appointment?

Abbie is wise not to panic, but she should see her doctor right away. Even though her last mammogram was clear, she needs to know that mammograms miss about 10 percent of breast cancers. And the farther apart mammograms are spaced, the greater the likelihood of a cancer coming up and growing in between those checkups. That's why doctors recommend annual mammograms.

But what about all those other patients ahead of you who don't seem all that sick? Can you speed up getting your own care by moaning and clutching your belly? Or will you die of heart failure while waiting for someone to have their hay fever treated?

No, say experts. Most ERs have a triage system to take vital signs and gauge the severity of patients' symptoms. Once you've been evaluated, let your condition speak for itself, advises Dr. Wynn. If you have a sore throat, you're going to wait. If you have a bleeding artery, you're not going to wait.

Still, you don't have to merely take a number.

Of course, a lump doesn't necessarily mean cancer. Abbie's lump could be a cyst, and if it's a simple cyst, nothing more needs to be done. We can usually make that diagnosis without operating, using needle biopsies in conjunction with a mammogram and ultrasound. Most of the time, lumps like Abbie's are benign, but the only way to know for sure is to get a tissue diagnosis or at least a diagnostic work-up.

If it is cancer, the advances we've made in diagnosis and treatment give Abbie a very good chance of being cured. But if she continues "watching it" for too long, she'll be in danger. If it's a tumor and she delays treatment, she runs the risk that as it gets bigger, it could shed tumor cells and spread to other parts of the body. And she could end up needing additional treatment beyond surgery, possibly chemotherapy and radiation.

Abbie shouldn't panic about the possibility of breast cancer, but she should seek medical help soon.

Expert consulted
Eva Singletary, M.D.
Chief of surgical breast service
University of Texas M. D. Anderson Cancer
*   Center*
Houston

If you've been waiting for what seems like an exceptionally long time, check back at the triage desk, suggests Deborah E. Trautman, R.N., director of nursing in the department of emergency medicine at Johns Hopkins Hospital in Baltimore.

Your Psychological Edge

If there's any good news about rushing to the ER, it's gender. Women, according to one psychologist, tend not to postpone treatment as much as men do. "Women are more socialized to ask for help than men are," notes Ellyn

Kaschak, Ph.D., professor of psychology at San José State University in California, lecturer, and author of *Engendered Lives*.

"No one wants to think they might be hauled into the emergency room, but that's not the time to educate yourself about dealing with doctors," she says. "Remember, you're the best expert on your own body."

In Case of Emergency

If you do end up in the ER, your sense of control doesn't have to end at the door. Here's what experts advise to help you handle your ER visit.

Tell them where it hurts. The more specific the better: where and how do you hurt? Is the pain sharp, dull, burning? Does anything make the pain better or worse? For example, if you've injured your ankle, does standing on it make the pain unbearable? Also, keep track of how long the pain has occurred and if it is intermittent or persistent, adds Trautman.

Rate your pain. On a scale of 1 to 10, 10 being the worst pain you've ever had, is that sharp stab a 10 or a 5? "What feels severe to you and me may be different," says Trautman, "but when you rate it, I can put it into perspective."

Getting worse? Get vocal. If you're in the waiting room with stomach pain and you suddenly want to lose your lunch, let the triage staff know, urges Dr. Bontempo. Any change in your condition could get you reevaluated and maybe seen faster.

Take a buddy. Call your spouse, friend, neighbor—just call on someone, advises Trautman. You'll need help to dig out your insurance card, write down medication instructions, and get home.

Keep the crowd down. Limit your emergency companions to two. Only one visitor may be allowed in your treatment area, anyway. And you won't have an entourage taking up patient space, notes Dr. Bontempo.

When to See Your Doctor

When is your doctor's waiting room a better choice than the ER's? It depends. What separates an emergency from a less critical condition isn't clear cut, notes Trautman, except for the ABCs. "Life-threatening emergencies are clearly anything to do with interrupting your Airway, Breathing, or Circulation," she says.

The following common symptoms aren't emergencies but call for professional care soon, suggests Dr. Wynn.

Drops of blood in the toilet. If bright red drops appear after a bowel movement, or there's blood on the toilet paper, chances are that it's a fissure or a hemorrhoid. There's also a chance, though, of an inflammation or colon cancer.

New or changed mole. Has a familiar mole gotten bigger, changed color or outline, or begun bleeding? Has a new one appeared? It should be checked for skin cancer cells.

Lingering cut. A cut or blister that doesn't heal in a month or two could point to diabetes or hardening of the arteries.

PART TWO

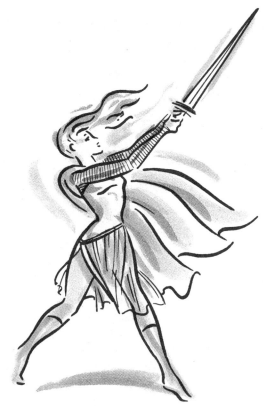

Engaging
the Enemy

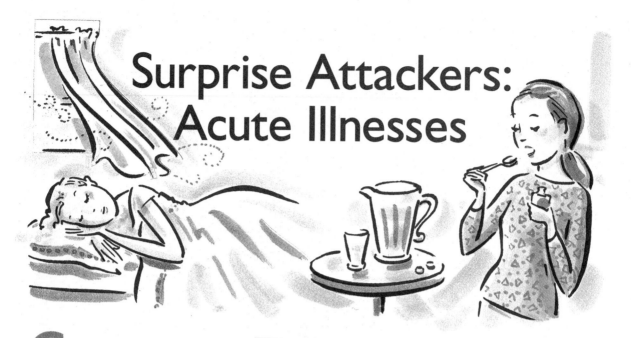

Surprise Attackers: Acute Illnesses

Caroline Saucer, 36, an editor from Old-wick, New Jersey, learned the meaning of "acute illness" the hard way. For some time, she had been having a pain that she suspected was caused by gallstones. Usually, it would come and go, but one particular night was different. Instead of easing off after a couple of hours, the pain grew worse. "It was like a knife right under my sternum," she says. By the time dawn arrived, she was exhausted and desperate. She called a friend to drive her to the hospital. "I'd had enough. I would never go through another night like that," she says.

Doctors told her they couldn't be certain that her lentil-size gallstones were the real culprits behind her pain, but after her gallbladder was removed, her discomfort went away. Four days after the surgery, she was back at work.

Anatomy of an Acute Illness

A gallbladder attack is typical of an acute illness. It comes on suddenly and tends to have a short and relatively severe course. All sorts of illnesses can come on suddenly, including infec-

tions, some cancers, food poisoning, aneurysms, strokes, pneumonia, ectopic pregnancies, shingles, severe allergic reactions, intestinal blockages, pelvic inflammatory disease, pancreatitis, perforated ulcers, blood clots, and kidney stones. Episodes of acute illness can also occur with a long-lasting chronic disease, says Susan Dunmire, M.D., associate professor of emergency medicine at the University of Pittsburgh Medical Center. "You can have heart disease for many years, but a heart attack is considered an acute illness," she says. "And asthma, diabetes, Crohn's disease, multiple sclerosis, and rheumatoid arthritis can all precipitate acute episodes."

Because there are so many different kinds of acute illnesses, the symptoms can vary tremendously. Pain is often a symptom, sometimes the worse pain you've ever had in your life, sometimes pain that wakes you up out of sleep. But some acute illnesses can be completely painless. If you've had a brain injury, such as a stroke, your only symptoms might be an altered level of consciousness or loss of function of an arm or leg. Fever is often a signal that you have a serious infection, but adults sometimes take awhile to build up to an alarmingly high fever.

"Symptoms can vary, but it eventually becomes clear to most people or members of their family that something is very wrong and that you need to see a doctor," Dr. Dunmire says.

Know What You Can Control

When the time comes, you may end up in an emergency room, or you may end up seeing your doctor in her office. Either way, it's hard to be entirely prepared. But there are things that you can do ahead of time to make your experience a little easier.

Know your doctor. "One of the best forms of 'protection' in the event of acute illness is an ongoing relationship with a primary-care doctor who knows your medical history and family history of illness," Dr. Dunmire says. "If you have a doctor you see regularly, call up and get advice about what to do." Make sure that your doctor and her staff understand clearly that you consider this an urgent matter and that you believe you need to be seen that day. Even if your doctor tells you to get to an emergency room, she can still be available to the emergency room staff by phone to provide them with important information.

Write a living will. It's an unfortunate fact of life that some acute illnesses have the potential to take a sudden turn for the worse. If you've

WOMEN ASK WHY

Why do they always say to drink plenty of fluids and get lots of rest when I'm feeling sick?

Water is an essential component of health. It's involved in every biochemical process in your body. And getting enough is particularly important when you're sick. Feverish sweating can dry you out, which can lead to dehydration and may drive up your fever. Throwing up or diarrhea can also dehydrate you. If you're taking drugs for your illness, drinking plenty of fluids helps to keep the toxic by-products of drug metabolism from reaching high concentrations in your kidneys and liver.

Water also helps to thin mucus so that you can cough it up or blow it out, which is important because trapped, thick mucus can promote secondary bacterial infections such as pneumonia.

Why do you need to rest? First of all, fighting off infection can be very fatiguing, and you'll need to rest just to keep up your strength. But there's another benefit to spending time in bed when you're ill. During sleep, your body secretes growth hormone, a powerful tissue healer. Lack of sleep, on the other hand, results in higher levels of stress hormones and a drop in immune function. So if you can't stay in bed around the clock while you're sick, get at least 8 hours of sleep a night and give yourself up to 2 weeks to ease back into your normal routine. You'll bounce back faster.

Expert consulted
Susan Dunmire, M.D.
Associate professor of emergency medicine
University of Pittsburgh Medical Center

been living for years with a chronic condition that occasionally turns nasty, you've probably thought about what you would want if, heaven forbid, your condition left you in a coma and requiring life support, such as a respirator. You can outline your wishes with a living will.

GREAT WAYS TO STAY OUT
OF THE EMERGENCY ROOM

Acute illness isn't the only reason that people end up in emergency rooms. An injury from an accident can get you there just as fast, says Susan Dunmire, M.D., associate professor of emergency medicine at the University of Pittsburgh Medical Center. Here are some things that you can easily do to prevent your chances of being injured.

- When you're in a car, always wear your seat belt.
- Never mix alcohol and driving, boating, biking, swimming, or using power tools. And don't get into a car that's being driven by someone who has been drinking.
- Always wear a helmet when your activity calls for it.
- Get enough sleep, and don't drive when you're sleepy.
- Store and label household chemicals properly. Keep them out of the reach of children.
- If you're the chief cook and bottle washer in your family, know how to handle food safely. That goes double for meat, especially ground meat. And remember that when cooking any kind of meat, pink is out and brown is in. Keep knives sharp so that they don't slip. Make sure that hands and knife handles are dry.
- Avoid ladder mishaps. Place the ladder's feet 1 foot out for every 4 feet up, and allow 3 feet of the ladder to extend above the top of the roof line. Never stand on the top two rungs.
- Avoid using space heaters. If you must use them, turn them off when you leave the house or go to sleep.

Keep copies with your doctor and with a close relative who will make decisions for you if you're unable. To get a copy of a living will that you can adapt to your needs, write to the Partnership for Caring: America's Voices for the Dying, 475 Riverside Drive, Room 1852, New York, NY 10115. The wills are available at minimal cost.

Buddy up. It's very helpful to have a trusted family member or friend accompany you to the doctor or hospital, says Robin Rudic, a social worker at the University of Pittsburgh Medical Center. "If you're very sick or very upset, it may be hard for you to communicate with the hospital staff about what is going on. A family member can help," she says.

Don't get separated. People can become anxious if they're separated from family members. Rudic says that it's perfectly legitimate to request that you and your family member remain together as much as possible. You may be separated during an initial evaluation or critical care, but you should be able to stay close the rest of the time.

Balance patience and demands. People often feel out of control when an acute illness strikes, and they want to be seen quickly and get answers fast, Rudic says.

While it is reasonable to expect to be seen quickly in an emergency room—within 20 minutes, depending on the severity of your symptoms—sometimes the answers don't come as fast as anyone would like, Dr. Dunmire says. "Especially for something like acute abdominal pain, it could be so many things that we can't get to the bottom of it immediately. Immediate, life-threatening problems are looked for first, but if none is apparent, sometimes the only thing a doctor can tell a patient is that her pain is not being caused by anything life-threatening and that the answer may come down the road with more testing."

"People can get very demanding and angry because they are afraid and have lost control," adds Rudic, "but a certain amount of patience is warranted in all this."

Life after an Acute Illness

Once the crisis is over, you may still have some recovering to do, Dr. Dunmire says. So seeing your doctor for follow-up care is important. If you've had a severe asthma attack, for instance, you may need to spend some time figuring out a medication routine that will prevent similar attacks in the future. If you've had a heart attack, you'll need dietary and exercise advice.

Your life can change quickly, drastically, and even permanently as a result of acute illness or injury. But whatever your situation, you can make the most of it. "I encourage people to do everything they can to get as well as they can," Rudic says. "Some people will need rehabilitation to recover, and many benefit from joining a support group." People who've had head trauma or spinal cord injuries, in particular, may need ongoing support to cope with their new way of life. Rudic points out that finding a balance between doing for yourself and getting the help you need can allow you to continue to get the most out of your life.

Prepare for Sudden Invasion: Seasonal Health

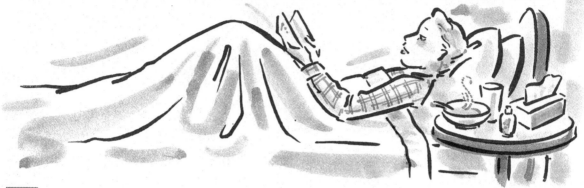

The common cold costs the American economy 15 million days in lost work every year. Influenza drives the number even higher. So what? If you have a cold or the flu right now, you want relief, not statistics.

Unfortunately, as everyone knows, there is no way to cure a cold or influenza once you're infected. But there are steps that you can take to help your body cope and heal as quickly as possible. Better yet, there are strategies that you can use to avoid coming down with these illnesses altogether.

Risk Factors

The most obvious risk factor for catching the cold or flu is exposure to the germs that cause it, but that doesn't necessarily mean standing in the direct line of fire of a sneeze or cough, says Carlene Muto, M.D., director of infection control and epidemiology in the division of infectious diseases at the University of Pittsburgh Medical Center. Although both diseases can be transmitted through the air, colds are actually more likely to be spread by touch. "All you need to do is touch something that someone sick touched or coughed on or sneezed on, then touch your own face, nose, or mouth," she says.

Time of year is also a risk factor. Colds and flu have a season, and it's fall/winter, says Dr. Muto. That's because in cold weather you spend more time indoors, in close quarters, and have more opportunity to be infected with germs and to infect others.

The rhinovirus (a virus that can cause the common cold) has a season that actually peaks in September and early October. The start of a new school year may be another contributing factor, as respiratory illness is more easily spread in the classroom and then is brought home to the other members of the family.

Some researchers also believe that your menstrual cycle, allergies that affect your nose and throat, and emotional stress can all make you more liable to catch a cold.

People with weakened immunity due to some other illness, poor nutrition, stress, or smoking are not at an increased risk of viral exposure; however, once exposed to a cold or flu virus, their bodies may be less capable of fighting off the infection, Dr. Muto says. Some types of respiratory allergies can also alter the mucous membranes in the nose and throat, making you more vulnerable to viral infections.

On the other hand, it's also true that if you've just had a cold, you're less likely to pick up another one right away. We're exposed to more than 100 types of cold viruses, and each type is distinct. Once you've had one of them, you develop an immunity to that particular virus that lasts about 2 years. You also develop a generalized immunity that protects you against the other 99 cold viruses for about a month.

Prevention

The steps to prevent colds and flu are simple and effective, but they require that you be vigilant, break old habits, and create new ones.

Flee from sneezers. Stay away from people who are coughing and sneezing. If you can't avoid them altogether, try not to get too close, and make your visits as brief as possible.

Wash up. Often, that rids your hands of any nasty viruses that may be waiting for a ride up to your nose or mouth.

Put your hands down. To make doubly sure that no cold or flu germs find their way into your body, keep your hands away from your face even after you have washed.

WOMEN ASK WHY

Why can't you get Lyme disease from a regular tick—and what's a deer tick, anyway?

*B*orrelia burgdorferi, the spiral-shaped organism that transmits Lyme disease, can move from a tick's midgut to its salivary glands in only two species: the deer tick in the Northeast and Midwest and the Pacific tick in the Northwest. Once the organism is in the tick's salivary glands, it can be injected into the bloodstream of whatever the tick snacks on—animals and humans. In general, the tick has to be attached for 36 to 48 hours before the Lyme disease organism is transmitted. So you have some time to remove the tick while your risk of getting Lyme disease remains low.

A deer tick is smaller than the common dog tick, the kind you're most likely to recognize. In its nymph stage, the deer tick is the size of a poppy seed. When it is engorged with blood, however, it can blow up to five times this size. An adult deer tick is about the size of a sesame seed and can get as big as a Raisinet after sucking your blood for a few days.

It can be difficult to tell an engorged deer tick from a regular tick. If you've been bitten, you may want to save the tick and ask someone from your local health department to identify the species. Most doctors do not prescribe antibiotics for a deer tick bite unless you develop symptoms of Lyme disease—skin rash around the site, headache, fever, stiff neck, aches and pains, and fatigue. If you are pregnant when you are bitten, however, prophylactic antibiotics are prescribed. A vaccine is recommended for people living in areas with a high prevalence of Lyme disease. It requires three shots: two given a month apart, usually in April and May, and one given a year after the first shot.

Expert consulted
Clarita E. Herrera, M.D.
Clinical instructor in primary care
New York Medical College
Valhalla

Disinfect. Three hours—that's how long rhinoviruses can live on surfaces outside a human body. Scrubbing those surfaces down with a virus-killing disinfectant may help stop the spread of disease.

Take a shot. Getting your annual flu vaccination shot is one of the nicest things that you can do for yourself. So do it.

Take a good multivitamin. So many vitamins and minerals are involved in proper immunity that it's a mistake to zero in on some and neglect the others, says Rachel Wissner, M.D., a family practitioner in Baton Rouge, Louisiana. A good multi will cover your bases.

Chew less fat. Fats, especially polyunsaturated fats, tend to suppress the immune system. Cut your total fat intake to 25 percent or less of your daily calories, says Dr. Wissner.

Destress—or else. Long-term psychological stress can inhibit many aspects of the immune response, including natural killer cell activity, T cell response, and antibody production. If you're getting lots of colds, you may need to consider stress as a factor, experts say.

There are lots of ways to reduce stress—exercise, meditation, breathing exercises. The trick is to find a balance that works well for you. It's not so surprising that the same nutrients that help ward off colds and flu, such as vitamins C and E and zinc, play a role in the body's production of stress hormones and in the hormones that help keep you relaxed.

HOW TO USE A THERMOMETER

What is a normal temperature for one person may not be quite the same for another, says Clarita E. Herrera, M.D., clinical instructor in primary care at New York Medical College in Valhalla. Generally speaking, a normal oral reading would be about 98.6°F. Rectal readings usually run a degree higher, at 99.6°; and axillary (or armpit) readings run 0.5 to 1 degree lower than oral.

Mercury thermometers used to be considered the gold standard, the most accurate, for taking a temperature, but digital thermometers now work just as well and are safer since they don't break.

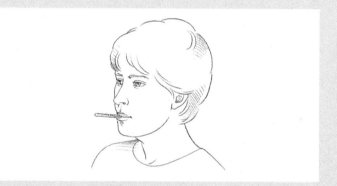

To use a mercury thermometer, shake it down, using quick flicks of your wrist, until it reads less than 96°F. Place the bulb under your tongue, just to one side of the center. Keep your lips closed; breathe through your nose. (If you have a stuffy nose, you can take a rectal or underarm temperature instead.) Leave the thermometer in place for 4 minutes.

Digital thermometers are safe, accurate, and fast. Look for one that claims to be accurate to within at least 0.2 degree. Some are accurate within 0.02 degree, but these may be a little more expensive. With most digital types, readings are obtained within a minute. The temperature is displayed much like the numbers on digital wristwatches.

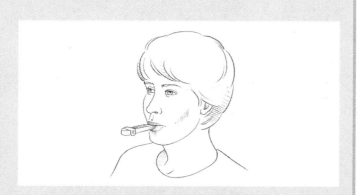

The digital thermometer can be used under the tongue, in the rectum, or in the armpit. Since turning the thermometer off clears the display, you do not need to shake it down beforehand. Usually, a beep or series of beeps indicates that the reading is done.

Ear (infrared) thermometers are accurate, quick, and relatively comfortable, but using one correctly requires some training. Follow package instructions carefully. The temperature is taken by placing the small cone-shaped end of the thermometer in the ear canal. The thermometer usually gives a reading within seconds.

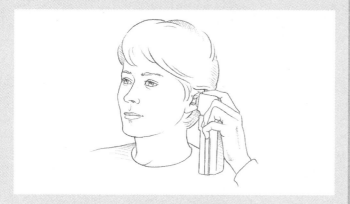

Heat given off by the eardrum and surrounding tissue is used to calculate body temperature. The thermometer converts the temperature to an oral or rectal reading and displays it on a digital screen.

Signs and Symptoms

Cold symptoms usually start 2 to 3 days after you have been infected, and include a sore throat, cough, headache, sneezing, and a clogged, runny nose. You may also have a slight fever of less than 100°F.

Flu symptoms usually appear within 2 to 4 days of your being infected. You're likely to have a headache, chills, and a dry cough, followed by body aches, fever, nasal congestion, and sore throat. The flu is highly contagious, and you can spread the virus for another 3 to 4 days after your symptoms appear.

Who Do I See?

Colds are a leading cause of visits to the family doctor, and people frequently receive antibiotics for colds when they do not need them. Colds are caused by viruses, not bacteria, and antibiotics won't faze them. "Sometimes, though, a cold can lead to a secondary bacterial infection of the middle ear or sinuses, in which case antibiotics may be in order," says Dr. Muto. "A high fever, shortness of breath, significantly swollen glands, severe facial pain in the sinuses, or a persistent cough that produces mucus all suggest you may have more than a simple cold and should see a doctor soon."

What Can I Expect?

Cold symptoms can last from 2 to 14 days, but two-thirds of all people infected recover in a week.

Flu viruses, on the other hand, have a whole-body effect that can leave you feeling tired for weeks. Give yourself up to 2 weeks to ease back into your normal routine. You will bounce back faster than if you push yourself, Dr. Muto says.

Conventional Wisdom

Many conventional doctors will tell you that there's not much they can do for you when you have a cold except advise you to get lots of rest and drink plenty of fluids. As for chicken soup, it actually may help. Sipping hot broth helps keep protective mucous layers in your nose and throat flowing, which in turn flushes away cold virus particles.

Here's what else traditional doctors suggest.

Take your pharmaceuticals. If you are coming down with the flu, you can take prescription antiviral drugs such as amantadine HCL (Symmetrel) or rimantadine HCL (Flumadine). If started within 2 days of symptoms, antiviral drugs can decrease the severity of symptoms and the duration of a bout of the flu. These drugs, however, work for only one kind of flu, called Type A.

Instead, your doctor may recommend a prescription powder inhaled through the mouth, called zanamivir (Relenza). In a study, this drug reduced the duration of a bout of the flu by a day or two. It also cut the chance of catching the flu by 72 percent. This drug works for two types of flu, A and B. A pill form of the flu antiviral drug oseltamivir (Tamiflu) is also available by prescription.

Use a humidifier. Dry air dries out your nasal membranes, making them less resistant to

Women Ask Why

Do I really have to get a flu shot every year?

Getting a flu shot is one of the best bargains in medicine. It really can protect you from getting the flu, and in a worst-case scenario, it might just save your life.

The influenza vaccine is actually a killed virus or a mix of viruses, and it works by making your immune system develop antibodies. So if and when your body becomes exposed to the virus, those antibodies are set to attack. Additionally, the antibody-producing part of your immune system actually has a memory. So if it has made antibodies against a particular virus once and is exposed to the same virus again, it can crank up production much faster the second time. It's almost as though it had the template already made.

Each year, a vaccine is made for whatever strains are most likely to strike, based on analyses of flu outbreaks around the world.

Vaccination is recommended for all people age 65 or older and people of any age with chronic diseases of the heart, lung, or kidneys; diabetes; compromised immune systems; or

attack from viruses. Keep your air humidity at 35 to 45 percent, Dr. Muto recommends. Indoor air-conditioning can be just as drying as heat, so you'll want to adjust your cooling system as well. If you're congested at night, keep a vaporizer at your bedside to get a direct shot of moist air.

Great Alternatives

There are hundreds of self-care herbal and nutritional remedies that can minimize the symptoms of a cold or flu, help you recover energy faster, and ward off future infections. "The

severe forms of anemia or asthma. It is also recommended for people who live in nursing homes or other places where people with chronic medical conditions live, for health-care workers, and for people who live in a household with a person who fits into any of these categories. Also, children or teenagers receiving long-term aspirin therapy, who therefore may be at risk for developing Reye's syndrome after a flu infection, should get vaccinated, as should women who will be in the second or third trimester of pregnancy during the flu season (which is November to April, making September through mid-November the best time to get the vaccine).

Most people don't have any side effects from a flu shot, but some feel soreness at the shot spot or develop a headache and slight fever for about a day after the vaccination.

A flu vaccine in the form of a nasal spray rather than a shot is expected to be available for the 2001–2002 flu season. The preventive whiff may eventually prove more protective than a shot.

Expert consulted
Clarita E. Herrera, M.D.
Clinical instructor in primary care
New York Medical College
Valhalla

trick is to pick the ones that work best for you, given your symptoms," says Jasmine Carino, N.D., a naturopathic physician with the Canadian College of Naturopathic Medicine in Toronto. Here are the details.

Don't skimp on the vitamin C. You need to take 1,000 to 3,000 milligrams a day of vitamin C to reduce your cold symptoms, Dr. Carino says. "You want to increase your dosage until you begin to have loose stools, then back off a bit." In studies that used this range of dosages, cold symptoms and durations were reduced by about 30 percent. Doses under 1,000 milligrams were ineffective.

Take 250 to 500 milligrams every few hours as soon as you are aware that a cold is coming on, and continue taking it for a few days more, even if your symptoms start to wane.

If you've had kidney stones or gallstones, take a smaller dose, up to 1,000 milligrams a day.

Add echinacea. "Of dozens of herbs used to treat colds and flu, echinacea, or purple coneflower, is one of the best," says Dr. Carino. Echinacea contains a diverse array of active components that stimulate different functions of the immune system to mount a response to a virus or bacteria.

Here again, it's best to start taking echinacea at the first signs of a cold or flu. How much you take depends on the severity of your symptoms. For the worst colds, take $\frac{1}{2}$ to 1 teaspoon of a liquid form (tincture or extract) every 2 hours. As symptoms improve, gradually decrease the dosage and frequency to $\frac{1}{4}$ teaspoon three times a day, Dr. Carino says.

Don't use echinacea if you're allergic to closely related plants, such ragweed, asters, and chrysanthemums. Don't use it if you have tuberculosis or an autoimmune condition, such as lupus or multiple sclerosis.

Suck on zinc. You may be able to cut your symptoms of sore throat, coughing, and nasal congestion from 8 to 4 days if you use zinc gluconate tablets or lozenges, according to a study done at the Cleveland Clinic. How much do you need to do the trick? In the Cleveland study, participants took a daily average of 4 to 8 lozenges containing 13.3 milligrams of zinc. This dose was effective. Possible side effects are nausea and a bad residual taste. Zinc's effectiveness in relieving cold symptoms is controversial.

STREP THROAT

Streptococci bacteria are nothing to fool around with. Strep throat infections range from mild to severe. In severe cases, fever, chills, headache, and abdominal pain may occur. Strep can simply invade your throat, causing severe pain, or it can become deadly, moving into your bloodstream where the poisons it produces can cause toxic shock syndrome or lead to heart or kidney damage.

Strep throat is spread just like colds and flu, through contact with someone infected with the bug. Children often bring it home and sometimes infect other family members. Symptoms usually appear 1 to 3 days after exposure and include painful, red tonsils or throat; a fever; swollen lymph glands in your neck; and, sometimes, white dots of pus on your tonsils or the back of your throat.

It's hard to tell just by looking at your throat whether you have strep or some other throat infection. "Even doctors can diagnose accurately with visual inspection only about 60 percent of the time," says Berrylin Ferguson, M.D., associate professor of otolaryngology at the University of Pittsburgh Medical Center. That's why they vigorously swab the back of the throat to do a culture for bacteria to confirm a diagnosis of strep throat. Sometimes, however, if strep is a suspect, your doctor will simply give you antibiotics. A 10-day course of penicillin is the usual treatment, and it's important to take the drug all 10 days, even if your sore throat is soon gone.

Inhale herbal vapors. Throw a teaspoon of dried basil, thyme, or oregano into a pot of steaming hot water and inhale the steam for a few minutes to unplug your sinuses and soothe your mucous membranes, Dr. Carino says. "It's great. Both have menthol properties that aid decongestion." For safe steaming, remove the pot from the stove and place it on a stable, heat-resistant surface. Drape a towel over your head and shoulders to enclose steam. Keep your face at least 12 inches from the water to avoid burns.

Get your body moving. Moderate exercise is an immune booster. It takes about a half-hour of aerobic exercise to sweep back into circulation white blood cells—key immune system components—that are stuck in your blood vessel walls. Studies also show that the number of certain immune system cells increases, at least temporarily, following exercise. Ideally, you should get a half-hour of aerobic exercise 5 days a week.

If you are actually coming down with something, listen to your body and pay attention to your symptoms, Dr. Carino says. Some people find that exercise makes them feel better, especially if it makes them sweat; others feel they need to rest.

Allow yourself to run a bit of a fever. Your fever is there for a purpose—to help your immune system destroy the enemy. An adult can safely run a fever of up to 102°F for a day or two while fighting a cold, Dr. Carino says. Support your body during this time by drinking lots of fluids and by resting.

Zinc is thought to help stop viral replication or to prevent viruses from entering cells in this application.

Take zinc lozenges as you feel a sore throat or cold coming on and for up to 2 days after you have recuperated, Dr. Carino says. You can find zinc gluconate lozenges at drugstores.

Hold the sugar. Sugar inhibits phagocytosis, the process by which viruses and bacteria are engulfed and then destroyed by white blood cells, says Dr. Carino.

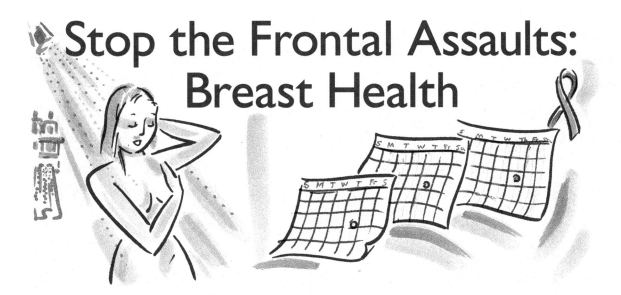

Stop the Frontal Assaults: Breast Health

Our breasts are not getting the attention they deserve.

Hard to imagine, isn't it? Female breasts seem so important in our culture. They're ogled, glorified, and vilified. They're displayed in the movies, accentuated in clothing design, and used to sell products. When Brandi Chastain, a defender for the U.S. women's national soccer team, hammered the game-winning shot past the Chinese goalie in the finals of the 1999 Women's World Cup, then joyously ripped off her jersey, they even made the news. Sometimes, it's easy to wish they weren't the focus of so much attention.

But there remains one kind of attention that they absolutely need and don't always get. Incredibly, even in this age of tremendous public awareness of breast cancer, some women still shrug off self-exams, mammograms, and other important screening tests.

"There is this unfortunate idea that if my breasts aren't causing me problems in my day-to-day life, if they're not causing me pain, then I don't need to get them examined regularly. Unfortunately, breast cancer doesn't bother most women until it's at a fairly advanced stage," says A. Marilyn Leitch, M.D., a surgical oncologist and professor of surgery at the University of Texas Southwestern Medical Center at Dallas.

That's why vigilance and early detection play such important roles in the battle against breast cancer.

Risk Factors

Few other places in the world have rates of breast cancer higher than those in the United States. Other than skin cancer, it is the most common form of malignancy diagnosed among women in this country, affecting 175,000 of us and claiming 43,000 lives each year. Only lung cancer is more lethal. Since 1973, the number of breast cancers diagnosed has increased about 2 percent annually, although much of that increase is the result of better methods of detection.

Doctors aren't certain what makes the breast so susceptible to cancer, but a number of factors are known to increase a woman's risk of developing the disease, including the following.

Age. The risk of breast cancer increases gradually as a woman gets older. It is rarely diagnosed in women under age 35, but all women age 40 and over are at increased risk. Most cases occur in women over age 50, and the risk is particularly high among women over age 60.

Family history. If your mother, sister, daughter, or at least two other close relatives, such as cousins, have a history of breast cancer, especially at an early age, you may be at high risk yourself, says Dr. Leitch. When checking your history, don't neglect your father's family. Even if he hasn't had the disease himself, if his mother or sister had it, he may carry a breast cancer gene. Risk assessment and genetic testing may be appropriate if you have a significant history of breast cancer on either side of your family.

Certain breast changes. A previous diagnosis of benign conditions or more than two breast biopsies are associated with a higher risk of cancer.

Late childbearing. Women who had their first children after the age of 30 have a greater chance of developing breast cancer than women who had children at a younger age.

Estrogen exposure. Women who began menstruating before age 12, experienced menopause after age 55, never had children, or took birth control pills or hormone-replacement therapy for a number of years may also be at higher risk. That's because these factors increase the amount of time that a woman's body is exposed to estrogen. And the longer you are exposed to estrogen, the more likely you are to develop breast cancer.

Risk factors are important, but paying too much attention to them may be misleading, as the odds that any one of them will trigger breast

STOPPING THE TIME BOMB: PREVENTIVE MASTECTOMY

Tricia Marrapodi knew it was only a matter of time. Her mother had died of breast cancer at the age of 44. Although Tricia was just 17 when it happened, she decided what she wanted. She would have a preventive mastectomy—her breast tissue would be surgically removed and replaced with saline implants, significantly reducing her chances of developing breast cancer. But a doctor persuaded her to wait until she was 30. By then, he told her, she would be better prepared both physically and emotionally for the ordeal.

So Tricia waited. Then, at age 27, her twin sister, Kelly Munsell, told Tricia that she had found a lump in her breast. A month later, Kelly underwent a mastectomy and began chemotherapy treatments for her cancer. Because she and Kelly are identical twins, Tricia's doctor estimated that her chances of developing breast cancer were more than 90 percent. Tricia knew the time had come. She had a double mastectomy at age 28.

"I feel I made the best decision, because of the peace of mind it has given me," Tricia says. "I still have a 2 percent chance of getting breast cancer because I still have some residual breast tissue. But my high risk before surgery had been a terrifying prospect. I feel as if a heavy burden has been lifted from my shoulders."

cancer is less than 1 percent, says Deborah Capko, M.D., breast surgeon and associate medical director of the Institute for Breast Care at Hackensack University Medical Center in New Jersey. In fact, many women with known risk factors do not get breast cancer. And many women who have none of these factors develop the disease. Doctors are hard-pressed to explain this paradox. That's why diligence is so critical.

"Most women who don't have a family history of breast cancer feel that they can let self-exams and mammograms slide a bit because they're not at risk," Dr. Capko says. "The truth is that most

Even though researchers have found that prophylactic mastectomies can reduce a woman's chance of getting breast cancer by up to 90 percent, most doctors consider this kind of surgery a radical option—even for women who have a long family history of the disease or who carry one of the two genes known to promote breast cancer.

"If we're going to do such drastic surgery, we want to be sure that the risk of developing breast cancer is very significant and high," says A. Marilyn Leitch, M.D., a surgical oncologist and professor of surgery at the University of Texas Southwestern Medical Center in Dallas. "So for somebody who is going to have a bilateral preventive mastectomy, my preference is for them to go through genetic testing and counseling."

But preemptive mastectomies aren't just for healthy women at risk. Some who have had cancer in one breast opt to have the other one removed as well.

"Once a woman has experienced breast cancer, she knows what is involved with the surgery and its effects. If she makes the decision, after careful thought, that she wants to have a preventive surgery on the other breast, then we will do that," Dr. Leitch says. "But we don't do that surgery very cavalierly. We do it only after a lot of thought and counseling."

women who get breast cancer do not have a family history or any of the other risk factors."

Prevention

There are no known surefire ways to prevent breast cancer, Dr. Capko says. But the following steps may help slash your risk.

Slim down. Weight control is one of the few modifiable lifestyle factors that may reduce a woman's risk of breast cancer, Dr. Capko says. Researchers suspect that excessive weight—more than 20 percent above your ideal range—sparks increased production of sex hormones that are thought to promote breast tumors. So if you're overweight, try shedding a few pounds. In fact, just trimming 150 calories per meal—the equivalent of a slice of cheese pizza, five gingersnaps, or a $\frac{1}{2}$-cup serving of vanilla ice cream—and eating one fewer snack per day can help you begin losing up to a pound a week. That may not sound like much, but in 6 months, you'll be nearly 24 pounds lighter, says Maria Simonson, Sc.D., Ph.D., director of the Health, Weight, and Stress Clinic at the Johns Hopkins Medical Institutions in Baltimore. Trimming visible fat off meats can save you about 60 calories per meal. Over a year, that can add up to 22,000 calories—and about $6\frac{1}{2}$ pounds that you don't have to worry about gaining.

Run for your life. Regular exercise, such as walking, swimming, gardening, or vigorously doing housework several times a week, can dramatically slash your risk of breast cancer even if you start late in life.

When researchers at the Mayo Clinic followed 1,806 postmenopausal women (whose average age was 75) for 11 years, they found that those who were moderately active had a 50 percent lower risk of breast cancer compared to sedentary women. Previous studies among those 40 or younger found similar effects among premenopausal women.

Exercise probably diminishes your breasts' exposure to cancer-promoting hormones, especially estrogen, says Leslie Bernstein, Ph.D., professor of preventive medicine at the University of Southern California School of Medicine in Los Angeles. Based on these studies, she suggests that women of all ages include a regular exercise program of 30 to 40 minutes a day as part of a healthy lifestyle.

Milk it for all it's worth. Sip on a warm mug of 1% milk with ¼ teaspoon almond extract at bedtime, suggests Holly McCord, R.D., nutrition editor for *Prevention* magazine. Milk fat contains an intriguing substance known as conjugated linoleic acid that fights breast cancer cells in test tubes and animals.

Defy it with D. Women whose diets contain higher amounts of vitamin D appear to have less risk of breast cancer. To ensure that you get the recommended level, make a multivitamin a part of your daily routine, McCord suggests.

Tea up. Green tea brims with antioxidants that block cancer by preventing damage to DNA, a cell's blueprint for reproducing itself properly, says McCord. Tests suggest that one of these compounds, EGCG, is 100 times stronger than vitamin C and 25 times stronger than vitamin E at protecting DNA. Although tests are ongoing, green tea inhibits the formation of cancer cells in animals. And in Japan, where people routinely drink two to three cups a day, cancer is less common and generally occurs at a much older age than in the United States. Green tea and its extracts (sold in capsule form) are available at most health food stores.

Go fishing. Order salmon whenever you find it on a restaurant's menu, McCord suggests. Salmon is rich in omega-3 fats, and research suggests that women with higher tissue levels of omega-3's have lower rates of breast cancer.

Flip a veggie patty. Flavorful vegetable burgers and sausages are better main-course choices than meat because they don't form compounds called heterocyclic amines when cooked. These compounds may be a major reason why women who eat lots of red meat and well-done meat seem to get more breast cancer, McCord says.

Booze, you lose. Consuming more than two alcoholic drinks a day may elevate estrogen levels, promote cell division, and increase your risk of breast cancer, Dr. Capko says. So if you imbibe, don't overdo it. Drink no more than one 12-ounce bottle of beer, 4-ounce glass of wine, or 1-ounce shot of hard liquor daily.

Stay in touch. If you know the shape and texture of your breasts by sight and touch, you're more likely to detect changes. In fact, 90 percent of the time, breast masses are found through self-exams. That's why it's so important to *really* do a monthly self-exam and not just think about it, Dr. Capko says. Do it at the same time each month. If you are premenopausal, do it 5 to 7 days after your period ends. By that time, your hormones will have stabilized and you'll get a better sense of your breasts' natural size and shape.

Begin with a visual inspection, says Dr. Capko. Stand before a mirror with your hands at your sides. Raise your hands and clasp them behind your head. Look for any changes in the size or shape of your breasts as well as for nipple discharge, redness, puckering, or dimpling. Then, press your hands firmly on your hips with your shoulders and elbows pulled forward; again, look for any changes.

Following this visual exam, check your breasts by touch. It's important to follow a definite pattern to ensure that you examine yourself thoroughly for any lumps. You may want to do it in the shower with soapy water so that your hands slide smoothly, suggests Dr. Capko.

WOMEN ASK WHY

Why do mammograms have to hurt so darned much?

During a mammogram, the breast is compressed between an x-ray plate below and a plastic cover above. This flattens out the breast so that as much tissue as possible can be imaged. It may seem painful, but in the big scheme of things, relative to other procedures, I really don't think it's that uncomfortable. I think the discomfort has more to do with anxiety and with fear of the results.

I highly recommend that women go to a center where the technicians do nothing but mammograms. They tend to have a bit more expertise and compassion than people who do a variety of x-ray studies and only occasionally do mammograms. The technician is more likely to talk you through the procedure, answering your questions and addressing your concerns. That gives you more sense of control and involvement, and it personalizes your care.

If you are uncomfortable during the procedure, let the technician know, and she should try her best to work with you. If she doesn't, then I would ask for another technician or find somewhere else to have your mammograms done.

Another thing women can do to lessen their discomfort is to schedule their mammograms so that they occur sometime during the 10 days after their periods normally begin. The breasts seem to be less tender during that time, and there's no chance of pregnancy.

Expert consulted
Emily Conant, M.D.
Associate professor and chief of breast imaging
The Hospital of the University of Pennsylvania
Philadelphia

PERFORMING A BREAST SELF-EXAM

Follow a definite pattern during breast self-exams, and do them the same way every time so that you become familiar with the way your breasts feel. One of the basic examination patterns is a circular shape, in which you move your fingers from the outer portions of your breast toward the nipple using small circles. But there are other patterns to use. To examine your breasts with the vertical pattern, slide your hand up and down in vertical lines from one side of your breast to the other. To try the wedge pattern, start from the nipple and work your fingers out to the edge of your breast and then back toward the nipple again. Continue until you have gone around your entire breast.

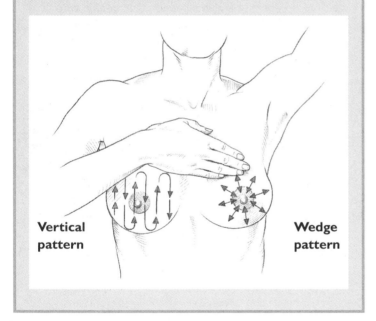

Vertical pattern

Wedge pattern

Squeeze it in. Even though you're not fond of the process, an annual mammogram after age 40 is one of the best ways to detect and get breast cancer treated in its earliest stages, Dr. Capko says.

Ask about tamoxifen. Ask your doctor to help you calculate your risk of developing breast cancer in the next 5 years (the National Cancer Institute offers computer programs that simplify this process). If your risk is at least 1.7 percent, which is considered a moderately high risk, ask your doctor about taking tamoxifen (Nolvadex), a drug that can cut your risk by 50 percent, Dr. Leitch suggests.

"For tamoxifen to be appropriate, the woman has to have a certain level of risk," Dr. Leitch says. "It's not something that a doctor would just give to any woman."

That's because there are some rare but significant risks associated with tamoxifen use, including potentially fatal side effects such as pulmonary embolism and uterine cancer. So be certain that you fully understand the pros and cons of this medication, given your level of risk for breast cancer, before taking it, recommends Dr. Leitch.

Signs and Symptoms

It can't be stated often enough: In its earliest and most treatable stages, breast cancer usually doesn't cause pain, and there may be no symptoms at all, so annual mammograms are extremely important. But sometimes, early symptoms do occur. The National Cancer Institute advises that you see your doctor if you notice any of the following:

- A lump or thickening in or near the breast or in the underarm area
- A change in the size or shape of the breast
- Nipple discharge or tenderness, or a nipple that has inverted back into the breast
- Ridges or pitting of the breast (the skin looks like the peel of an orange)

◆ A change in the way the skin of the breast, areola, or nipple looks or feels (for instance, warm, swollen, red, or scaly)

Don't Panic!

The vast majority of breast lumps are not cancerous, says Emily Conant, M.D., associate professor and chief of breast imaging at the Hospital of the University of Pennsylvania in Philadelphia. "More often than not, what you're feeling is an area of normal breast tissue or a benign lump," she says. Common benign causes of breast lumps include cysts, fibroadenomas, or areas of fibrosis. But don't let the medical names frighten you. These lumps are all harmless. Your doctor will probably conduct imaging tests, such as mammography or ultrasound. In some cases, a biopsy or a needle aspiration, which draws fluid out of the area of concern with a syringe, is necessary to confirm these benign diagnoses.

Even if the growth is cancerous, often the diagnosis is still hopeful, Dr. Leitch says. In fact, women now have more treatment options and hope for survival than ever before. Ninety-nine percent of women whose breast cancer is detected early are still alive 5 years after diagnosis, and 98 percent survive 10 years or more.

In addition, the death rate from breast cancer has tumbled in recent years. A woman's estimated lifetime risk for dying of breast cancer is less than 4 percent. In comparison, a woman's lifetime risk of dying of heart disease, stroke, di-

BREAST PAIN: WHAT DOES IT MEAN?

"Probably 70 to 75 percent of women experience breast pain at some point in their lives. Often, it's associated with hormonal changes that occur in the breast during the menstrual cycle. Many women also get breast pain in their forties as they approach menopause. Again, it's all due to hormones—they're completely out of control. You may have constant pain in the breast in the form of a feeling of fullness, burning, or throbbing. Hormonal influences on the breast are truly incredible," says Deborah Capko, M.D., breast surgeon and associate medical director of the Institute for Breast Care at Hackensack University Medical Center in New Jersey.

Cysts and mastitis, a painful condition usually associated with breastfeeding, also can trigger sensitivity and tenderness. Arthritic conditions in the ribs and sternum are other possible sources of breast pain. And medications such as birth control pills can cause pain. But breast pain, particularly if it correlates with your menstrual cycle, is rarely a symptom of breast cancer.

Certainly, keep track of your pain, record its comings and goings in a notebook, if you like, and mention it to your doctor, Dr. Capko says. But in most cases, warm compresses and over-the-counter pain relievers or anti-inflammatory medications such as acetaminophen or ibuprofen, used as directed on the label, will alleviate the problem.

abetes, or complications of osteoporosis hovers near 40 percent, Dr. Capko says.

If you're concerned about disfigurement, you should know that breast-conservation surgery has become an option in all but the most advanced cancers, Dr. Capko says. Even those women who have total mastectomies, or complete removals of the breasts, lymph nodes, and surrounding tissue, are often able to get immediate reconstructive surgery, helping to blunt the psychological blow of losing a natural breast.

Finally, rather than panicking, try as best

as you can to maintain a positive attitude, suggests Patricia Gordon, M.D., director of radiation oncology at the Century City Hospital in Los Angeles.

"Attitude plays an enormous role in one's ability to recover from breast cancer," Dr. Gordon says. "Mind over matter is extraordinarily important. Having a positive attitude, having a loving family, having a significant other all contribute to an enhancement of well-being. And a sense of well-being will help you through the process of treatment."

Who Do I See?

If you develop any suspicious signs or symptoms, start with your gynecologist, suggests Barbara Fowble, M.D., a radiation oncologist at Fox Chase Cancer Center in Philadelphia.

Keep in mind that benign lumps often feel different from cancerous ones. Some doctors examine the breast in only one position, which makes it more difficult for them to get a complete sense of size, shape, and texture of a suspicious lump. So when you go in for the breast exam, make sure that your doctor checks your breasts in at least two positions, such as lying down with your arms raised up over your head and then standing or sitting upright, Dr. Capko suggests.

What Can I Expect?

If, after a careful physical exam, your doctor suspects that there is something abnormal in your breast, she may order further tests such as a mammogram or an ultrasonogram, a test that

MY MAMA TOLD ME

Will standing too close to a microwave give me cancer?

Microwaves have really helped some people eat better on the run. From heating up last night's hearty leftovers to zapping a side of veggies to go along with that bagel, they've given women an extra minute to eat their more nutritious, quickly cooked meals.

And the meals *are* more nutritious. In addition to re-heating a healthy food item, microwaving can retain the vitamins and minerals in vegetables.

Yet, for all its advantages, microwaving still makes us a little nervous. Notice how we talk about "nuking" our food when we put it in that oven. So what's the story? Are those invisible rays harmful? And do the ovens leak?

Microwave ovens are designed to keep their energy waves enclosed. Although some people may be concerned that leaking microwaves could injure a person standing in front of an oven, that's highly unlikely. To be certain that your microwave oven is safe, check the seals around the door to be sure that they're intact and in good condition. If you can slide a piece of paper between the door and the oven, the seal has deteriorated, and you should have it re-

uses high-frequency sound waves to help determine if a lump is solid or fluid.

If those tests raise further suspicions, then your doctor may recommend that you have a biopsy. This can be done with a special needle, or the surgeon may opt to cut out all or part of the lump. A pathologist will examine the tissue under a microscope to check for cancer cells.

If it turns out to be cancer, there's a good chance that you'll be deluged by fear, anxiety, anger, and resentment. "Women's breasts are very important emotionally. After all, our society puts a lot of emphasis on a woman's breasts. So when you tell a woman that she has this cancer,

placed. If you're still concerned, have a repairman check it for you.

When using microwave ovens in your office or elsewhere, stand away from them while they're operating.

And, if you're concerned about microwaves' effect on foods—just what *is* going on with all those excited molecules?—minimize your concern by microwaving only in glass, ceramic, or microwaveable-plastic containers. Those old margarine tubs and plastic wrap may melt and possibly leach chemicals and other foreign molecules into your food. (Plastic wrap covering a dish or bowl but not touching the food is all right for trapping steam.)

There's also no evidence that food chemistry can be altered by microwaving. The truth is that a microwave oven is a useful appliance for reheating leftovers in appropriate microwaveable containers, heating microwaveable dinners in their specially designed packages, cooking some foods from scratch (oatmeal, vegetables, potatoes, or poached fish or chicken), or even making yourself a quick cup of herbal tea or hot cocoa.

Expert consulted
Barbara P. Klein, Ph.D.
Professor of food science and human nutrition
University of Illinois
Urbana-Champaign

she's thinking about all of the losses she faces: her breasts, her womanhood, her life," Dr. Capko says. "A lot of people might say, 'Oh look at the big picture. Your breast isn't that important; it's your life that matters.' It all goes together. I don't think it's fair to flippantly suggest, 'Oh, you need a mastectomy,' because the fear of losing a breast is overwhelming."

When a woman learns that she has breast cancer, her first response may be a desire for treatment, any treatment, immediately. Resist that impulse, Dr. Capko urges. Keep in mind that breast cancer is seldom a medical emergency. Your treatment options or odds of survival probably won't change if you take a few days to let the news sink in.

"What I tell a patient is, 'You're going to have questions. You're probably not going to understand fully what I've just told you. And there are a couple of things that you're going to start doing,'" Dr. Capko says. "'First, you're going to read everything you can about breast cancer. Second, you'll probably mention your diagnosis to a few close friends and family members. As soon as you do that, anybody you've ever known is going to call you with advice. They're going to tell you about the best doctor. They're going to call you with suggestions of all the things you need to do.'"

"So you really need to filter that information, educate yourself about the disease, and work with your doctor to determine the best course of action for you. And that's going to take some time."

Conventional Wisdom

Treatment will depend on the size of your tumor and whether it has spread to the lymph nodes or other parts of your body. But in general, your treatment will likely include surgery, radiation, chemotherapy, or various combinations of these cancer fighters, Dr. Capko says.

Breast cancer surgery dates back to medical antiquity and remains a fundamental treatment for the disease. But the days of automatically doing a total mastectomy are long past. A lumpectomy, removal of the tumor only, followed by radiation is far more likely now.

Radiation therapy, also called radiotherapy, uses high-energy rays to kill cancer cells and stop them from growing. Your doctors may also sug-

WHEN A LUMP ISN'T BREAST CANCER

Notify your doctor about any new lumps that you notice or feel in your breasts. Although cancer is always a possibility, in most cases, these lumps will be harmless. Here's a closer look at a couple of common noncancerous conditions that you may develop.

Benign fibroadenomas are firm, movable, fibrous breast lumps, of any size. These painless growths, which may feel like small, rubbery marbles and are firm to the touch, usually form from the fibrous supportive tissue of the breast. But they can also arise from the tissues in the mammary glands, the 15 to 20 milk reservoirs that radiate outward from the nipple. They most commonly occur in women before age 30 and may enlarge at certain times during the menstrual cycle. Although these lumps are harmless, most physicians will urge you to have them surgically removed—at least the first time they occur—to rule out cancer.

Fibrocystic breast disease is a condition in which numerous cysts form in both breasts, accompanied by lumpiness and breast pain. It usually affects women over 30 and dissipates after menopause. If you develop severe discomfort, your doctor may prescribe drugs such as tamoxifen (Nolvadex) to curb cyst formation. In addition, you may be able to ease the symptoms if you avoid consuming caffeine, alcohol, and saturated fats.

gest placing radioactive implants into your breast. In some cases, you may receive both types of treatment. Radiation therapy, alone or in conjunction with chemotherapy or hormonal therapy, may also be used before surgery to destroy cancer cells and shrink the tumor. Despite the effectiveness of radiation, some women are apprehensive about undergoing it, Dr. Capko says.

"They just have visions of what it can do to you," Dr. Capko says. "They don't understand that it is limited to the breast itself. They don't understand that the equipment that is used is very sophisticated and ensures that the radiation gets directly centered on the breast. They fear that receiving radiation will cause cancer somewhere else in the body. That's just not true."

In fact, the typical side effects of a 5-day-a-week, 6-week course of radiation may be limited to a sunburnlike burn on the treated breast, fatigue, and the loss of underarm hair near the treated breast, Dr. Fowble says.

Chemotherapy, which involves a combination of anti-cancer drugs, is a standard treatment for premenopausal women whose breast tumors are greater than 1 centimeter in diameter. Because these drugs travel throughout the bloodstream, they are often able to destroy cancerous tissue that other forms of treatment can't completely wipe out. It is also a treatment that scares many women because of its reputation for having nasty side effects, including hair loss, nausea, vomiting, and loss of appetite. But in many cases, these side effects can be controlled or even eliminated.

"Without question, we are making giant advances in the management of the side effects of cancer treatments. There are medications that counteract chemotherapy's side effects to the point that most women experience little or no nausea or vomiting," Dr. Gordon says.

In the future, there may be no need for surgery, radiation, or chemotherapy. In fact, researchers are working on a number of vaccines that may eradicate breast cancer and other forms of cancer.

Among the most promising is a vaccine developed by James McCoy, Ph.D., a former staff immunologist at the National Cancer Institute. Dr. McCoy's vaccine is autologous, meaning that it is made from a person's own cancer cells.

"It's not a preventive vaccine. It is a treatment," Dr. McCoy says.

The process begins when a surgeon removes a sample of the person's tumor, freezes it, and ships it to Dr. McCoy's laboratory in Atlanta. There, the specimen is used to create the vaccine. The initial treatment is given to individuals during a 2-week visit to the lab.

So far, the best results have occurred among people who have breast cancer. All of those women in Dr. McCoy's studies who have stage I and stage II breast cancer—two of the earliest stages of the disease—have been in remission for 5 years. In other words, they have no detectable signs of cancer and will likely stay that way.

"It looks as if when there isn't a large tumor present, the vaccine activates the immune system and keeps the cancer from recurring," Dr. McCoy says.

Although the vaccine is less effective against more advanced tumors, it also appears to help one in five of those women.

"I suspect that vaccines and genetic engineering are the ways that breast cancer is eventually going to be cured," Dr. Capko says.

Great Alternatives

Traditional Chinese medicine is a good complementary treatment for breast cancer and may

WOMEN ASK WHY

Why do men rarely get breast cancer?

Breast cancer is a disease most of us associate only with women. In fact, we are 100 times more likely than men to develop this disease. Our breasts are constantly being bombarded with estrogen and other hormones that can trigger tumor growth.

But it's important to remember that men have some breast tissue as well and occasionally can develop cancer there. In fact, about 1,300 men each year develop the disease. When men do get breast cancer, it often isn't detected until a later stage than it would be in women, simply because men aren't screened for it as vigilantly as we are.

It wouldn't be a bad idea for men to examine their breasts on a regular basis, just as they should be examining their testicles. Like women, men should also be aware of the warning signs of breast cancers, including a lump on or near the breast, bleeding from the nipple, and swollen lymph nodes under the arm. If they develop these symptoms, they should see a doctor as soon as possible.

Expert consulted
Emily Conant, M.D.
Associate professor and chief of breast imaging
The Hospital of the University of Pennsylvania
Philadelphia

help prevent the disease altogether, says Nan Lu, O.M.D., doctor of traditional Chinese medicine and founder of the Breast Cancer Prevention Project at the Traditional Chinese Medicine World Foundation in New York City.

According to traditional Chinese medicine, the root cause of breast cancer is the stagnation of vital energy, or *chi*, in the meridians (energy pathways) that run through the breast area, and the malfunction of one or more of three major organs—the kidney, stomach, and liver. This stagnation and dysfunction, explains Dr. Lu, are caused primarily by chronic negative emotional energy that has built up over time. In the view of ancient Chinese medical tradition, when energy stagnates over time, a small seed can progress to a cancerous mass.

"Chinese medicine has at least a 500-year history of dealing with breast cancer," says Dr. Lu, author of *Traditional Chinese Medicine: A Woman's Guide to Healing from Breast Cancer*. "As long as energy can flow freely through the meridians, and the five major organs—liver, heart, spleen, lung, and kidney—function in harmony, then a tumor can't form."

Practitioners of traditional Chinese medicine look for warning signs, such as the sudden appearance of red veins in the heels of the feet, that suggest energy flow in the body is blocked. If it is, you could be at risk for breast cancer until you get your *chi* back into balance.

Dr. Lu and other traditional Chinese healers use a variety of methods to balance *chi*, including acupuncture, acupressure, massage, herbs such as angelica root or Chinese ginseng, and *qigong*, a self-healing system that uses movements and postures to stimulate energy flow in the body.

"It can make your whole life change," Dr. Lu says. "It is not uncommon in China for women to recover from breast cancer by practicing *qigong*."

Foods such as broccoli, cauliflower, garlic, eggplant, mushrooms, pineapple, and watermelon can help improve the energy function of the liver—the major organ that controls women's health—and can help prevent breast cancer, Dr. Lu says.

For more information about traditional Chinese medicine and its role in preventing breast cancer or its recurrence, write to the Traditional Chinese Medicine World Foundation, 396 Broadway, #502, New York, NY 10013.

Protect Against the Enemy Within: Digestive Health

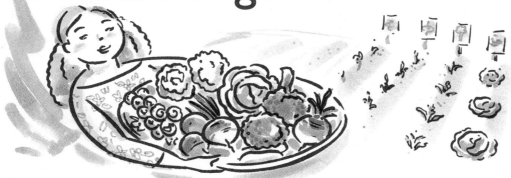

Audrey Hepburn died of cancer in 1993. You probably knew that. But do you know what type of cancer she had? Few people do, and it's no surprise. Bowel cancer isn't the sort of thing the media likes to mention, especially where beautiful, elegant, and charming women like Ms. Hepburn are concerned.

"We don't talk about colon cancer; it's unmentionable," says Mary Elizabeth Roth, M.D., clinical professor at Wayne State University in Southfield, Michigan, and a member of the American Cancer Society's Committee on Colon Cancer. Nevertheless, what needs to be mentioned about bowel tumors is both deadly serious and extremely hopeful.

The facts are that cancer of the colon and rectum (colorectal cancer) will kill some 56,600 people this year—almost half of them women. It is the second leading cause of cancer death in the United States. And it is highly preventable. "This is a cancer that no one needs to have," asserts Ernestine Hambrick, M.D., founder and chairperson of the Stop Colon/Rectal Cancer Foundation in Chicago.

Risk Factors

Often silent and symptomless, colorectal tumors grow either from the colon, which is the last 5 to 6 feet of your intestine, or from the rectum, which is the last 8 inches or so of your digestive tract.

As with many cancers, there are important factors in your life that can help determine your risk for getting this disease.

Age. As years pile up, so does your likelihood of developing colorectal cancer. In fact, the incidence is six times higher among those age 65 and older than among those ages 40 to 64.

Genetics. Some people are at greater risk if one of their parents or a sibling have had colorectal cancer or polyps.

Personal history. If you've already had colon cancer, colon polyps, or inflammatory bowel disease, your risk rises.

Diet. Can't get enough red meat? If you eat too much, you may be asking for trouble. It's full of saturated fats, which some research has suggested may raise your risk for colorectal cancer.

WOMAN TO WOMAN

She Survived a Bowel Tumor through Early Detection

Professionally, she's a registered nurse working at a cancer-screening center. But Kathy Lee, 45, of Voorhees, New Jersey, had very personal reasons to take action against colon cancer. Here's her story.

When my paternal uncle died of colon cancer in 1994, I had my first colonoscopy, a test that examines the large intestine (colon) with a flexible, lighted tube and a camera. There was nothing suspicious. When my father died 2 years later from complications of a different cancer test, I had another colonoscopy. This one revealed a small, malignant polyp.

By this time, I knew my family had a strong cancer connection: Colon cancer had taken two uncles, an aunt, my paternal grandfather, and my great-uncle. Because of this family history and my relatively young age (almost 42), my surgeon wanted to remove a large section of my colon because my risk of recurrence was high.

So I spent a day taking laxatives and antibiotics to clean out my colon. Then came the operation.

Although the tumor was small (less than ¾ inch) and was caught early, it had invaded the first layer of the colon wall. I found out I have hereditary non-polyposis colorectal cancer (HNPCC). It puts me, my brother, and my sister at high risk for a number of cancers, so I pushed my siblings into cancer screenings. They both had precancerous colon polyps removed.

A few months after the surgery, I started having nightmares—even when my 6-month check for new polyps showed nothing. And I felt guilty for surviving with "just" surgery and no chemotherapy or radiation treatments. Physically, the only symptom I have from my surgery is diarrhea.

Today, I'm just glad to be alive. I spend a lot of time communicating with other cancer survivors and new patients, even sharing my experience on the Web.

I wish more people knew that if colon cancer is detected early, they can beat it. Sure, the whole process of having your colon cleaned out, examined, and operated on is embarrassing, but you can't die of embarrassment.

Lack of exercise. Being overweight raises the danger.

Hormones. There's evidence that postmenopausal women on hormone-replacement therapy enjoy a lowered risk.

Aspirin. This nonsteroidal anti-inflammatory drug (NSAID) may stave off several digestive tract cancers, including colon cancer.

Prevention

Diet, a healthy lifestyle, and screening are the three keys to minimizing your chances of getting colon cancer. "We're increasing our health consciousness about eating less fat and more fiber," observes Ana Maria Lopez, M.D., assistant professor of clinical medicine at the Arizona Cancer Center at the University of Arizona College of Medicine in Tucson. She offers these guidelines for healthy living.

Favor fruits, veggies, and fiber. Get at least five servings of fruits and vegetables daily, plus at least 25 grams of fiber per day from high-fiber foods such as whole-grain breads.

Forgo fat. Limit high-fat foods, especially red meat (try for just one serving per week).

Fortify with folic acid. Most multivitamins contain the 400 micrograms daily that may lower risk of colorectal cancer.

Go easy on the alcohol. Because it may deplete the body's folate supply, women should limit drinks to one a day.

Don't smoke. Cigarettes may promote the cell changes that lead to colon cancer.

Work it out. Just 30 minutes of physical activity (walking, jogging, playing tennis) several days a week helps cut risk.

Get some added protection. Screening tests can detect the polyps, or grapelike growths, that sometimes turn into cancers. "You find the polyps, you take 'em out, you don't get cancer; it's that simple," sums up Dr. Hambrick, a former colorectal surgeon.

"If everybody over 50 got regular screenings, we could cut the colorectal cancer death rate in half," says Dr. Lopez.

The American Cancer Society recommends the following:

Digital rectal exam. The doctor inserts a lubricated, gloved finger into the rectum to feel for irregular or abnormal areas. This is performed before a sigmoidoscopy, colonoscopy, or double-contrast barium enema.

Fecal occult blood test (FOBT). This annual test looks for hidden ("occult") blood in stool samples. You take home a test kit to collect samples from three consecutive bowel movements and return the kit to a lab for evaluation.

Sigmoidoscopy. This is a visual exam inside the rectum and lower colon. With a flexible, lighted tube called a sigmoidoscope, a doctor looks inside the rectum and lower colon for cancer or polyps. New research suggests, though, that this exam misses some cancers. A sigmoidoscopy examines only the lower one-third and left side of the colon; colon cancers show up more often on the right side of the colon. No one is quite sure why.

MY MAMA TOLD ME

Will spicy food and coffee really give me ulcers?

This myth persists because some people do have problems with spicy food and coffee, but those problems aren't ulcers.

We have a muscle called the lower esophageal sphincter that keeps stomach contents from moving back up into the esophagus. Coffee contains caffeine and acid; spicy food has capsaicin, the "hot" element in hot peppers, and all these can relax the sphincter a bit. When that happens, some of your stomach contents back up into the esophagus, and you get the burning sensation in your chest that we call heartburn.

Many people assume that this heartburn feeling is related to ulcers because it mimics the kind of pain that comes from an ulcer in either the stomach or the duodenum (the first part of the small intestine).

So the answer is no to ulcers from spicy food and coffee, but yes to heartburn.

Expert consulted
Kim E. Barrett, Ph.D.
Professor of medicine
University of California, San Diego, School of Medicine

Colonoscopy. The advantage of a colonoscopy over a sigmoidoscopy is that the colonoscopy views the entire colon. After cleaning out the colon beforehand with a special diet and laxatives, you're sedated for this procedure: With a colonoscope (like a sigmoidoscope, but longer), a doctor examines the entire colon via a video camera and display. Polyps can be removed with a wire loop passed through the tube.

Double-contrast barium enema. With this procedure, done in a hospital or clinic, x-rays of the colon are taken after barium sulfate is injected through the rectum. As with a colonoscopy, a prior cleaning out of the bowel is necessary.

Following an initial normal barium enema result, the American Cancer Society recommends that everyone over 50 follow one of three screening options.

- ❥ A fecal occult blood test every year, plus a sigmoidoscopy every 5 years
- ❥ A colonoscopy every 10 years
- ❥ A double-contrast barium enema every 5 to 10 years

Follow the "rule of 10." For those with genetic or personal-history risk factors, more frequent screening that begins at a younger age is recommended. "Just as with breast cancer, it's important to look at your family history," advises Nancy E. Kemeny, M.D., attending physician of gastrointestinal oncology service at the Memorial Sloan-Kettering Cancer Center in New York City. If a parent had colon cancer before age 50, you should start screening when you're 10 years younger than that person's age when diagnosed. For example, if your mother had colon cancer at 40, start screening at 30.

Signs and Symptoms

The danger of this cancer is that it can appear silently, over a period of years, with no symptoms. But colorectal cancer can also announce itself in these ways, according Dr. Kemeny.

- ❥ Rectal bleeding
- ❥ Blood in the stool
- ❥ Change in bowel habits: constipation, diarrhea, or trouble having a complete bowel movement
- ❥ Cramping or stomach pain

Don't Panic!

While any of colon cancer's symptoms merit prompt medical attention, they don't necessarily signal the disease. Dr. Roth details some other conditions that can mimic the symptoms of this cancer.

Hemorrhoids. These dilated veins and swollen tissue at or near the anus can produce bleeding.

Leaking blood vessel. The technical term is angiodysplasia, and it means a blood vessel in the intestine has become fragile and bleeds.

Parasites. These unwelcome visitors can cause blood in the stool.

Antibiotics. Some of these medications can produce both blood in the stool and rectal bleeding.

Other bowel diseases. Rectal bleeding can also come from ulcerative colitis, which is an inflammation of the colon that causes ulcers, and Crohn's disease, a similar ailment. Diverticulitis, an advanced condition involving small pockets ballooning out from the colon, can also cause rectal bleeding as well as abdominal pain.

Who Do I See?

For two of the basic screening tests, you probably need go no farther than your primary-care physician's office. Both the FOBT and sigmoidoscopy can be performed in a doctor's office. The more revealing colonoscopy and barium enema require a hospital or clinic.

For a colonoscopy, you'll see a gastroenterologist, a doctor with expertise in the stomach and intestines. If a malignancy requiring removal of part of an organ or other body part is found, a surgeon will be called on. At the same time, according to Dr. Kemeny, a consultation with a tumor specialist, or oncologist, may occur.

INFLAMMATORY BOWEL DISEASE

There are bumps along the road in the digestive tracts of some one million Americans, and for the half who are female, the road gets rougher every month. These are the women who have ulcerative colitis and Crohn's disease, known together as inflammatory bowel disease (IBD).

The causes of both diseases are unknown. Short of colon surgery for ulcerative colitis, there's no known cure.

Both bring ulcers, or sores, to the digestive tract. Ulcerative colitis targets just the inner lining of the colon (large intestine) and the rectum, while Crohn's disease can strike anywhere from mouth to anus. The symptoms of both chronic ailments are distressing enough, but our hormone cycles can make things even worse.

"With ulcerative colitis and Crohn's, women can have symptoms other than bloody diarrhea, abdominal pain, constipation, or weight loss," notes Sunanda V. Kane, M.D., assistant professor of medicine at the University of Chicago. The two digestive ills can also make periods irregular, she says, and research indicates that they can also aggravate premenstrual woes.

Another factor is that ibuprofen or other nonsteroidal anti-inflammatory drugs used to ease menstrual aches can worsen IBD inflammation. That's why Dr. Kane looks to alternative means to ease monthly flare-ups.

Instead of steroids, which some doctors recommend but which Dr. Kane calls "the atom bomb" of anti-inflammatories, women's IBD flare-ups may be eased by willow bark, black cohosh, ginseng tea, chamomile tea, primrose oil, and extracts from red clover or yams. (Always check with your physician before taking any herb or supplement, she cautions.)

"There's evidence that these herbs help relax the smooth muscle around the colon, easing cramping and possibly diarrhea, too," relates Dr. Kane.

Prolonged steroid use is a known factor in bone loss, so women treated with steroidal drugs for IBD may be at especially high risk for osteoporosis when menopause brings a decrease in estrogen. Here, calcium supplements can help guard against bone loss; hormone-replacement therapy, as appropriate, may also help back up bones.

What Can I Expect?

If screening tests reveal tumors, the emotional impact can be as serious as the physical. "Women are shocked to find that they have colon cancer," says Nada L. Stotland, M.D., chairperson of psychiatry at the Illinois Masonic Medical Center in Chicago and editor of the book *Psychological Aspects of Women's Healthcare*.

Fear based on ignorance is one of the biggest challenges of the disease. "The colon is kind of 'dirty' and unknown; it's supposed to just do its work and not bother you," Dr. Stotland says. To overcome that fear and ignorance, she urges these steps.

Have an appointment pal. If you get a diagnosis of cancer, request a follow-up visit to which you can bring a friend or family member. "When somebody tells you bad news like this, you don't hear anything else," informs Dr. Stotland. Your companion may be better able to absorb and retain the details.

Put pen to paper. You won't remember all your questions for the doctor, says Dr. Stotland, so write them down beforehand.

Share strength in numbers. Find a cancer support group, urges Dr. Stotland, especially one led by a counseling professional; literature indicates that it makes a positive difference.

TRACT TREK: WHAT'S BEHIND YOUR BELLYACHE

It's tough to suffer through a bout of abdominal pain when you're not sure if last night's chili is to blame. Maybe it's appendicitis? Maybe a gallstone? Use this quick guide to see what may be behind your stomachache, and see a doctor if you suspect any of the following.

Upper-Right Quadrant

- Gallbladder. Gallstones' pain is very sharp after eating, then eases.
- Liver. Dull, crampy pain could be autoimmune hepatitis or other liver ills.
- Duodenum. A burning pain after meals could be a duodenal ulcer.

Between Breasts

- Stomach. Burning, sharp pain that eases with food may be a sign of stomach ulcer.
- Pancreas. Pancreatitis inflammation causes pain, fever, and nausea.

Upper-Left Quadrant

- Nothing gastrointestinal.

Lower-Right Quadrant

- Appendix. Pain in this region is probably appendicitis; in pregnancy after 6 months, appendix moves to upper-right quadrant.
- Cecum. This is the first part of colon; it rarely gets inflamed by itself.

Belly Button

- Ileum. A dull to very sharp pain 1 to 2 hours after eating could be Crohn's disease. Commonly misidentified as the stomach, it's the small intestine.

Conventional Wisdom

On the diagnostic side, "virtual colonoscopy" may make this invasive exam less so. With the aid of computed tomography scanning, in the future, you may not have to have an instrument actually inserted into your colon, notes Dr. Hambrick.

Colon cancer treatment means basically three

Lower-Left Quadrant

➤ Colon. Crampy pain could be diverticulitis. A variety of bowel disorders often bring a change in bowel habits.

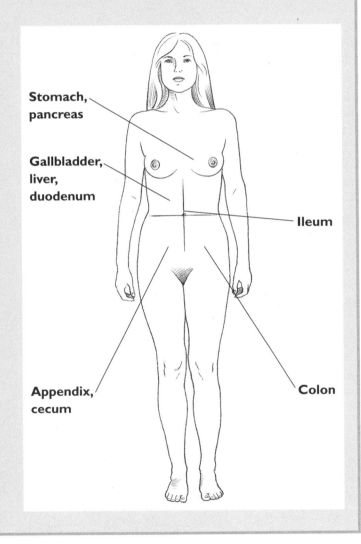

Stomach, pancreas

Gallbladder, liver, duodenum

Ileum

Appendix, cecum

Colon

they're going to get a colostomy, but that's very rare today," says Dr. Kemeny. A colostomy is an opening in the belly for eliminating body waste. Modern colon surgery removes the cancerous tumor, plus normal tissue on either side; the remaining portions of the colon are then reattached.

Often used with surgery, radiation therapy kills cancer cells with high-energy beams. Chemotherapy has traditionally concentrated on a drug called 5-FU (fluorouracil), but new companion drugs are emerging that give us a lot of new, effective options, says Dr Kemeny.

Great Alternatives

Diet, supplements, and herbs dominate the priority treatment list, according to alternative expert Irene Catania, N.D., a naturopathic physician in Ho-Ho-Kus, New Jersey, who has studied cancer therapies extensively. Emphasizing that her work with cancer patients is considered "adjunctive therapy," that is, designed to work along with traditional approaches, Dr. Catania offers these general strategies.

Make the move to veggies. A diet shift to mostly (if not all) vegetables is Dr. Catania's prime eating advice. Consume fresh produce, grains and legumes, plus six daily glasses of fresh veggie juices.

Go organic. When buying produce, shop for organic varieties, which don't contain pesticides that may aggravate cancer, says Dr. Catania.

Dish up fish. Fish oils and flaxseed oil can help balance cancer-fighting essential fatty

things: surgery, radiation therapy, and chemotherapy. Advances in surgery and drug treatments make the future more hopeful.

"People think that if they have colon cancer,

DIVERT DIVERTICULOSIS WITH BREAKFAST

Skipping breakfast can set a place at your body's "table" for one of the most common colon problems in the country: diverticulosis. In itself, it's relatively harmless, causing almost no symptoms except rectal bleeding. But it can lead to big trouble.

Often, the disease occurs with age. By 80, half of all Americans have it, but it can hit much earlier. If people don't have enough fiber in their diets, or have extra gas or insufficient stool volume, the natural weak spots in the wall of the colon can start to sag, says Sunanda V. Kane, M.D., assistant professor of medicine at the University of Chicago. This leads to "pouching" that from the outside of the colon looks like little mushrooms sprouting, explains Dr. Kane. Over time, the pouches can attract hard-to-digest items, like seeds or corn kernels, and become infected. At that point, diverticulosis becomes diverticulitis, a potentially serious inflammatory disease that can produce an emergency infection.

Our mothers told us that breakfast is the important meal of the day for a reason, affirms Dr. Kane. "When we put food in our stomachs, this signals the colon to evacuate and make room," she says. If a woman has a busy morning routine with little time for much except coffee, this reflex starts to shut down. The result is constipation.

So breakfast is the colon's cue to clear out. But what's in the breakfast is key. "If you develop diverticulosis younger than age 60, you're probably not dispelling gas enough, or not forming solid bowel movements," Dr. Kane says. The answer is more soluble fiber. Her advice:

Go for grains. Eat whole-grain breads and cereals and anything with wheat bran for a total of 25 to 30 grams of fiber daily.

Try the soluble solution. Insoluble fiber (in some over-the-counter "fiber" preparations) can only make things worse if your colon is already irritated. Pick the preparations that contain psyllium, starting with a tablespoon dissolved in 8 ounces of water daily, Dr. Kane advises.

Welcome water. It's nature's laxative, says Dr. Kane. The optimum dosage is eight 8-ounce glasses per day.

acids; aim for a minimum of 3,000 milligrams. Don't take fish oil if you have a bleeding disorder or uncontrolled high blood pressure, if you take anticoagulants (blood thinners) or use aspirin regularly, or if you are allergic to any kind of fish. People with diabetes should not take fish oil because of its high fat content. Fish oil increases bleeding time, possibly resulting in nosebleeds and easy bruising, and may cause upset stomach. Finally, do not substitute with fish-liver oil. It is high in vitamins A and D, which are toxic in large amounts.

Send in the supplements. Studies in Europe suggest that an antioxidant called reduced glutathione helps those on chemo- or radiation therapy cope better with side effects, says Dr. Catania. Reduced glutathione is used in very high doses, so Dr. Catania recommends that you consult with your health practitioner. She also recommends a high-quality multivitamin/mineral supplement.

Popular antioxidants like vitamins E and C and zinc are also on Dr. Catania's list.

Herbal arsenal. To deliver the benefits of different herbs, Dr. Catania often prescribes combinations or sequences of different ones. These include ginkgo, echinacea, astragalus, licorice, larch (from the tree), and maitake and shiitake mushrooms, all of which may help patients strengthen their immune systems.

Know Your Worst Enemy: Lung Health

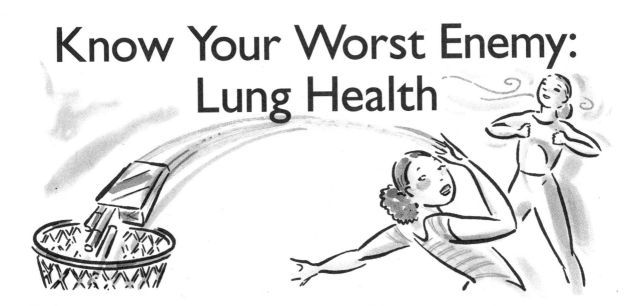

Lung cancer was a rare disease until the early 20th century. As late as 1912, there had been a total of only 374 reported cases of the disease, and the vast majority of those involved men. Although a few daring women smoked prior to World War I, we did not take up smoking in large numbers until the 1940s. Then, as lighting up became the norm rather than the exception, lung cancer rates among women skyrocketed. In 1987, lung cancer surpassed breast cancer as the leading cause of cancer deaths among women. By 1999, more than 42 percent of people who died of the disease were female. Each year in the United States, more than 77,000 women develop lung cancer, and about 68,000 die of it.

Risk Factors

Without a doubt, smoking is the number one risk factor for lung cancer. In fact, according to the Wyoming Department of Health, which has been monitoring all of Wyoming's cancer cases since 1962, the real seven warning signs of lung cancer are the cigarette-industry giants: U.S. Tobacco, Philip Morris, R. J. Reynolds, Brown & Williamson, Lorillard, British American Tobacco, and the Liggett Group.

The tragedy is that more than 90 percent of lung cancers among women could be prevented if we did just one thing: quit smoking. Each puff you inhale contains more than 4,000 compounds and at least 60 known cancer-causing agents, including substances used to make insecticide, rat poison, toilet bowl disinfectant, and embalming fluid. Tobacco smoke even contains hydrogen cyanide, a deadly poison used in prison gas chambers. If you smoke a pack or less a day, you are 7 times more likely to die of lung cancer than women who don't. If you smoke more than a pack a day, your risk of dying of lung cancer is a staggering 15 times higher than a nonsmoker's.

"Fifty percent of women who smoke are going to die of a smoking-related illness. Fifty percent. That's like flipping a coin. The odds are not good. I can't think of anything worse for your health that you could do in your life than smoking," says Linda Ford, M.D., past president of the American Lung Association.

Women Ask Why

Why doesn't my family doctor ever recommend vitamins and herbs when I'm feeling sick?

Unfortunately, most medical training overlooks the use of vitamins and herbs to treat illness. Physicians are trained in evidence-based medicine. That means when they treat a disease, they use procedures and medications that have been rigorously studied and that have good track records of evidence showing that they are effective in treating a specific ailment.

Until recently, herbal remedies have been subjected to few scientifically rigorous studies. Although more data is available on vitamin-and-mineral therapy (such as vitamin D and calcium for osteoporosis, or zinc for a sore throat), it has yet to become part of core medical studies. Additionally, a lack of regulation of vitamins and herbal products exists. Even when your physician prescribes these therapies, she cannot ensure what these products actually contain. I believe that as more studies become available, you will quickly see vitamins and herbs finding their way into mainstream medicine.

Expert consulted
Jan I. Maby, D.O.
Medical director
Cobble Hill Health Center
Brooklyn, New York

Granted, some women who have never taken a puff in their lives and are in the best of shape, such as Kim Perrot of the WNBA Houston Comets, do get lung cancer, but those cases are extremely rare. In most instances, nonsmokers who develop lung cancer have a long history of exposure to secondhand, or sidestream, smoke either in their workplaces or at home. Most of the chemicals that are found in mainstream smoke are also found in sidestream smoke and have the same cancer-promoting effects. In fact, each year about 3,000 people die of lung cancer as a result of breathing the smoke of other people's cigarettes.

Radon, a naturally occurring gas produced by the radioactive decay of uranium in the soil and water, has been linked to about 10,000 deaths from lung cancer annually. Statistically, it is the second most common cause of the disease. But in reality, many physicians suspect that smoking is probably a major contributor even in those cases.

"People like to blame anything else but smoking for their lung problems," Dr. Ford says. "'No, it's not the smoking I've been doing for the last 40 years that caused my cancer, it's the radon in my basement!' Very few lung cancers are caused by radon alone."

Prevention

Quit, quit, quit! Make it your mantra. Make it your obsession. Make it happen, Dr. Ford says.

"Sometimes, people have to stand up for themselves and say, 'Okay, I was foolish to start. I am addicted, but I can do something about it,'" Dr. Ford says. "You empower yourself to make that first step, which is always the hardest one. You will probably start and stop, start and stop, start and stop many times before you finally quit. That's okay. Don't feel too bad if you don't make it the first few times. Keep your eye on the goal, and the

MY MAMA TOLD ME

Does smoking really stunt your growth?

First of all, smoking will almost certainly stunt your life expectancy. In fact, smokers live an average of 7 years less than nonsmokers. It will also very likely stunt the quality of your life as you get older, since emphysema, chronic bronchitis, and other respiratory problems associated with smoking will make doing daily chores and activities difficult. So yes, in an indirect way smoking does stunt your growth.

Smoking increases your risk of osteoporosis, a disease whose name literally means "holes in the bones." It occurs when the loss of bone tissue exceeds its replacement. A silent disease, osteoporosis robs bones of their strength over time, particularly in the years following menopause. Osteoporosis can cause the bones in your spine to crack and fracture and can make you appear as if you have lost height.

But if you stop smoking—and it is never too late to do that—and begin exercising and taking calcium and vitamin D, you actually can reverse some of the effects of this disease. So osteoporosis is yet another reason not to ever smoke if you haven't started, and to quit if you have.

Expert consulted
Jan I. Maby, D.O.
Medical director
Cobble Hill Health Center
Brooklyn, New York

goal is quitting—living completely tobacco-free."

Certainly, it may be difficult, but it is never too late to stop and allow your body to repair the harm you've done to it, says Antoinette Wozniak, M.D., a clinical oncologist at the Barbara Ann Karmanos Cancer Institute in Detroit. Within 8 hours after your last cigarette, the oxygen levels in your blood will increase and the levels of carbon monoxide will plummet. In 48 hours, the final traces of nicotine will leave your body, and your ability to taste and smell will be enhanced. In 72 hours, your lung capacity will increase, and you'll breathe easier because your bronchial tubes will have relaxed. Within a week, virtually all the harmful chemicals produced by smoking will have left your body. In less than 3 months, your lung function will have improved 30 percent. Within 9 months, any residual coughing, fatigue, and shortness of breath will have dissipated. Your lungs will have increased their ability to cleanse themselves, remove excess mucus, and fend off infections.

And in just 10 years after lighting up for the last time, your risk of dying of lung cancer will be about the same as that of a woman who has never smoked.

Quitting, of course, is simple in theory—just throw your cigarettes out—but often difficult in practice. That's because nicotine, the prime ingredient in tobacco, is one of the most addictive substances known. Once you're in its grasp, it takes a determined effort to break free, particularly if you've been smoking for a number of years and you are a woman.

Women apparently metabolize nicotine more slowly than men, says Robert Klesges, Ph.D., a smoking-cessation expert at the University of Memphis and coauthor of *How Women Can Fi-*

Pneumonia

Women who smoke more than 20 cigarettes a day are three times more likely to develop pneumonia than women who have never taken a puff.

Even if you smoke less than that, your risk of pneumonia is still greater than a nonsmoker's, says Monica Kraft, M.D., a pulmonologist and assistant professor of medicine at the National Jewish Medical and Research Center in Denver. That's because women who smoke have fewer cilia, the hairlike cells that help clear bacteria, viruses, and other invaders out of their lungs. "Cigarette smoke actually paralyzes the cilia. So you've lost an important defense mechanism right there," she says. In addition, smoking disrupts the work of macrophages, immune cells that normally surround and destroy the dangerous particles that attack your lungs.

The net result is an increased risk of pneumonia. Pneumonia develops when phlegm, fluid, and other debris clog your airways and fill the air sacs in your lungs. This accumulation interferes with your lungs' normal ability to remove carbon dioxide from your body and deliver life-giving oxygen to your blood and tissues. Viral pneumonia is more contagious but usually less severe than bacterial pneumonia. Its symptoms include gradual appetite loss, slowly rising fever, muscle soreness, and a dry, unproductive cough that can develop into a phlegm-producing cough over several days.

Bacterial pneumonia, such as Legionnaires' disease, is far more dangerous and usually causes more violent symptoms than viral pneumonia. Unlike viral pneumonia, bacterial forms of the disease can be treated with antibiotics.

The best thing that you can do to prevent pneumonia is to quit smoking, Dr. Kraft says. In addition, an annual flu shot and a pneumonia vaccine every 5 years can help keep this disease caged. If you develop chills, fever, headache, fatigue, chest pain, or a productive cough, consult your physician, Dr. Kraft urges. If you are diagnosed with pneumonia, drink plenty of fluids (at least eight 8-ounce glasses of water daily), get lots of rest, and finish any medication that your doctor prescribes for you. In addition, keep coughing—although it may be painful, it will help clear phlegm out of your lungs and speed your recovery.

nally Stop Smoking. This means that cigarette for cigarette, women may have higher levels of nicotine in their bodies and, therefore, may be more dependent on the drug than men are. So when a woman tries to quit, her withdrawal symptoms may be more intense.

Then, there's the weight issue. Fear of weight gain after quitting is far more common among women than among men. In fact, it is probably the single biggest difference between why women and men smoke, according to Dr. Klesges. The truth is that the average weight gain for women who quit is about 13 pounds. It isn't inevitable, however, that you will gain weight. Once you nip your smoking in the bud, you can focus on your weight. So despite the barriers, you can quit once and for all. Here's how you can get started.

Stay in sync. Timing is everything if you're a premenopausal woman trying to quit. Plan to stop smoking at the end of your period (the beginning of your menstrual cycle) because you'll experience fewer and less intense withdrawal symptoms, Dr. Klesges suggests.

Set a quit date. Women (and men, for that matter) who set a definite day to quit and stick to it are more likely to stop smoking than those who don't. Avoid picking stressful holidays like New Year's Day or Thanksgiving, and don't select a date that is weeks or months away. Odds are that your resolve to quit will evaporate by then, Dr. Klesges says.

Cut back. Since women metabolize nicotine more slowly than men do, gradually cutting down may be a better way for you to quit than going cold turkey, Dr. Klesges says. Pick situations and places where you won't smoke, such as in the car, on the telephone, or in the kitchen. Or, you can try rationing your cigarettes. Carry only enough smokes with you to reach your limit for that day. If you normally smoke a pack daily, plan on cutting back to 15 cigarettes a day by the end of the first week, 10 cigarettes by the end of the second week, and none by the end of the third week.

Toss those weeds. The night before you quit, go through a quitting ritual, Dr. Klesges suggests. Throw out all of your tobacco products. Don't hold back. Lighters? Matches? Ashtrays? Pitch them. If you have any hidden stashes in places like pockets or glove compartments, toss those as well.

Can the cups. Women who smoke are more likely to drink coffee, tea, and other caffeinated beverages, Dr. Klesges says. Laying off tobacco increases caffeine's stimulating effects in your body. So if you are trying to quit smoking, you should cut your caffeine consumption in half. Otherwise, you may feel more jittery and start craving a smoke.

Make a pact. Team up with a friend. Research suggests that social support helps women—but not men—quit smoking. Hook up with a pal who is as committed to quitting as you are. It's a bad sign, for instance, if the person says, "Yeah, I guess I could give it a

---

PLEURISY

Some things in life just naturally go together. Spaghetti and meatballs. Pearls and basic black. Lucy and Ethel. And less pleasantly, pneumonia and pleurisy.

"Pleurisy is a common scenario with pneumonia. They tend to go together," says Monica Kraft, M.D., a pulmonologist and assistant professor of medicine at the National Jewish Medical and Research Center in Denver.

Pleurisy is an inflammation of the thin, transparent membrane called the pleura that covers your lungs and lines the inside of your chest wall. Usually caused by a viral or bacterial infection, this inflammation triggers breathing difficulties and can lead to extreme chest pain. It can precede pneumonia and is often an early warning sign of the disease, Dr. Kraft says.

Less commonly, acute bronchitis or a pulmonary embolism, which is a blood clot in your arteries leading to your lungs, can cause pleurisy.

Over-the-counter analgesics such as acetaminophen or ibuprofen, when used as directed, can help ease your chest pain, Dr. Kraft says. But remember that this is a temporary solution. Any chest pain should be evaluated by a doctor as soon as possible.

---

try." If you get that kind of tepid response, ask someone else to join your crusade, Dr. Klesges says. If your spouse smokes and refuses to quit when you do, frankly, it will be more difficult for you to stop. At the very least, ask him not to smoke inside your home or in your presence.

Stick to a plan. Once you find someone who is as committed to quitting as you are, the two of you should:

➧ Speak to each other every day. Frequent, daily contact is crucial, especially in the early stages of quitting. After you both quit, agree that you will call each other—even if it is 3 o'clock in the morning—if either of you is tempted to have a cigarette, Dr. Klesges says.

◆ Remain positive. Don't gripe or complain. Focus on the goal and how you can help each other stay on track.

◆ Support your buddy even if you are having a rough time. Don't let her down. Offer plenty of encouragement such as, "Yes, withdrawal symptoms are tough, but let's think of ways to help you past them."

◆ Think of your cravings and other withdrawal symptoms as challenges that you can overcome together.

Chew, stick, or swallow. When used as directed, over-the-counter products such as nicotine gum and patches as well as prescription medications such as bupropion (Zyban) can help lessen your urges to smoke, Dr. Klesges says. But keep in mind that these products are only a partial solution. They work best when used in conjunction with a formalized smoking-cessation program.

Keep it outside. If you are exposed to secondhand smoke on a regular basis, ask the smokers in your household to puff away outdoors. Suggest to your guests that they go outside if they wish to smoke at your house, Dr. Ford suggests. "The harder it is for a smoker to smoke, the less they will smoke—which is more healthy for them as well."

Keep radon out, too. The combination of smoking and radon exposure more than doubles your risk of developing lung cancer. So in addition to stamping out your tobacco habit, check up on the radon levels in your home, Dr. Ford suggests. Get a radon detector, available at many hardware stores, and place it in the basement or the lowest living areas of your home. Since radon levels can fluctuate daily, get a detector that will measure radon levels for at least 6 months. When the detector has completed its

task, mail the device to a laboratory that analyzes the data and then sends you a report.

Radon is measured in units called picocuries per liter. If your test results are greater than 4 picocuries per liter, the highest exposure recommended by the Environmental Protection Agency, then you should consider ways to fix the problem, such as sealing large cracks in your basement with caulk, installing a venting pipe to the roof, or simply using a window fan to flush the radon out.

Get a scan. If you smoke or are a former smoker, a painless 20-second test could save your life by detecting lung cancer at an early, curable stage, says Claudia I. Henschke, M.D., Ph.D., professor of radiology and division chief of chest imaging at the New York Weill Cornell Center of New York Presbyterian Hospital in New York City.

In her study of 1,000 smokers and former smokers age 60 and older, Dr. Henschke found that low-radiation-dose computed tomography (CT scan) can detect lung tumors long before they appear on chest x-rays. Dr. Henschke and her team found 23 early-stage lung cancers among these people. Only 4 of those tumors were visible on chest x-rays, the standard diagnostic imaging technique. Traditionally, lung cancer tumors have been about the size of oranges when they are discovered. But the CT scan found tumors that were no bigger than grains of rice.

"Lung cancer is deadly because we never had a good way to find it early. Now we do," Dr. Henschke says. "CT screening transforms the prognosis for lung cancer, just as mammography did for breast cancer. The current 5-year survival rate for lung cancer is only 14 percent. But that could soar to 80 percent if all smokers and ex-smokers received annual CT exams and early treatment." So ask your doctor about annual CT screening for lung cancer.

Signs and Symptoms

A persistent cough is the most common symptom of lung cancer.

"A lot of smokers have a nagging cough. Many pass it off as a smoker's cough. But they may also tell you that it's a different kind of cough than they've ever had before. It is either more productive or constant," says Dr. Wozniak.

So see your doctor if you notice a persistent cough or any change in your smoker's hack, particularly if you cough up blood. In addition, be wary of the following symptoms, according to Dr. Wozniak: suddenly developing shortness of breath during routine activities, such as climbing stairs, that haven't caused breathing difficulties in the past; wheezing; hoarseness; constant chest, shoulder, or arm pain; frequent bouts of pneumonia or bronchitis; unexplained weight loss; persistent fatigue; or swelling in your face, neck, or upper chest.

Don't Panic!

Acute bronchitis also may cause a persistent cough, shortness of breath, chest pain, and bloody sputum. You also may have pneumonia or a lung abscess—a pus-laden sac of dead tissue that forms as your body fights off an infection. Or you may have a more serious condition, such as emphysema or tuberculosis.

The important thing, says Dr. Wozniak, is to

SHACKLE YOUR CRAVINGS

If you are overwhelmed by a cigarette craving, you can still prevent a full-blown relapse if you follow these guidelines, says Robert Klesges, Ph.D., a smoking-cessation expert at the University of Memphis and coauthor of *How Women Can Finally Stop Smoking*.

- Never bum a smoke or accept a cigarette that is offered to you. Most women who relapse didn't purchase their cigarettes. They asked other smokers for them. Don't fall into this trap.

- Force yourself to go out and get the cigarettes yourself. If you're in a bar, for instance, don't purchase a pack from a vending machine in the lobby. Leave. Walk or drive to a convenience store or supermarket. Even then, allow 10 minutes to pass before you make your purchase. First, it will get you away from the sights, sounds, and other cues that are fueling your craving. Second, it will give you time to think about whether smoking is really what you want to do again. And third, since most cravings pass within a couple of minutes, odds are that you'll decide against the purchase.

- If you do purchase a pack, smoke one—in a place other than where you were originally tempted—then throw the rest of the pack away. If you want another one, repeat the process: Buy a new pack, smoke one, and throw the rest away. Most women who have cravings just want to smoke one, not an entire pack. If you keep the pack after smoking one, you'll be more tempted to smoke the rest plus a lot more.

If you do completely relapse, don't dwell on your setback. Set a new quit date right away and stick to it, Dr. Klesges urges.

---

see your doctor as soon as possible if you notice any of the warning signs, because the earlier a cancer is detected, the better your chances of survival.

"The worst thing that women can do is to take on the ostrich position with their heads buried in the sand," Dr. Wozniak says. "They panic, thinking that maybe these symptoms will just go away. But by the time they finally pull their heads out of the ground, it may be several months later, and they may be beyond what we can reasonably deal with."

Who Do I See?

If you experience lung discomfort, pay a visit to your family doctor first. "Most pulmonary complaints can be handled by primary-care practitioners," says Lisa Bellini, M.D., assistant professor of medicine in the pulmonary, allergy, and critical-care division at the University of Pennsylvania Medical Center in Philadelphia. If your primary-care practitioner suspects a problem, she may decide to consult a pulmonologist for a second opinion.

If an x-ray reveals a lung mass, you will probably be referred to a pulmonologist, who will evaluate whether or not the mass is cancerous. "If your primary-care physician has already made the diagnosis, you can see either a pulmonologist, who will test to see to what stage the tumor has advanced, or an oncologist," says Dr. Bellini.

What Can I Expect?

If your doctor suspects that you have lung cancer, she will likely order several tests to confirm the diagnosis. If you have a productive cough, for instance, your doctor will probably have your sputum screened for cancer cells. Your doctor also may order a chest x-ray or a CT scan. In addition, she may insert a small tube called a bronchoscope through your nose or mouth, down your throat, and into your bronchial tubes. During this procedure, your doctor will likely collect a sample of lung tissue so that it can be examined under a microscope for cancer cells. A biopsy also may be done during a mediastinoscopy, a procedure in which a scope is inserted into your chest through a small incision.

If the sample is cancerous, these tests also will help your physician determine what type of lung cancer you have and how far it has spread.

"The first thing that lung cancer patients fear is dying. And when they think about the treatment, they get totally scared. They worry about getting sick from the treatment or losing their hair. They worry about the cost," says Ritsuko Komaki, M.D., a radiation oncologist at the University of Texas M. D. Anderson Cancer Center in Houston. "They often express a lot of anger. They'll think, 'So-and-so has smoked just as long as I have, and she doesn't have lung cancer. Why me?'"

Conventional Wisdom

Treatment will depend on a number of factors, including the size and location of the cancer and whether or not it has spread to your lymph nodes or other organs. According to one estimate, 5 to 10 years elapse between the development of the first lung cancer cell and diagnosis of the disease. Because lung cancer is symptomless during much of its growth, three out of every four lung tumors have spread elsewhere prior to diagnosis and can't be cured by surgery alone.

Often, treatment will include a combination of surgery, radiation therapy, and chemotherapy.

The best thing you can do for yourself after diagnosis—if you haven't done it already—is quit smoking, Dr. Komaki says. Nicotine increases your body's use of energy and literally siphons off nutrients that could help you fight the disease.

"There is plenty of evidence that if a person continues to smoke after a diagnosis of lung cancer, the outcome is much worse compared to that of a person who does quit. If you continue to smoke—even if the first lung cancer is treatable—your risk of a second lung cancer or head-and-neck cancer in the next few years is greatly increased," adds Dr. Komaki.

Great Alternatives

In her book *Herbs for Health and Healing*, Kathi Keville, director of the American Herb Association, suggests that a "withdrawal" tincture made from fresh oats can help a smoker break the habit. To try it, combine 1 teaspoon tincture (or glycerite) of fresh oat berries, ½ teaspoon each of tinctures of valerian rhizome and skullcap leaves, and ½ teaspoon each of tinctures of St. John's wort leaves and passionflower. Keep the combination in a 1- to 2-ounce amber or dark-blue glass bottle with a dropper lid, and take 2 to 5 dropperfuls each day. All of these ingredients are available at most health food stores.

While the herbs in this formula are generally considered safe, some could cause problems for certain people. If you have celiac disease (a gluten intolerance), do not use oat berries. Do not use valerian with sleep-enhancing or mood-regulating medications. It may also cause heart palpitations and nervousness—if so, discontinue use. Do not use St. John's wort with antidepressants without your doctor's approval, and avoid overexposure to direct sunlight while taking it.

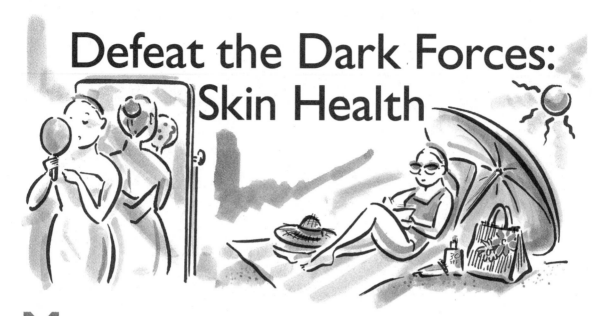

Defeat the Dark Forces: Skin Health

Melanoma is the seventh most common cancer among women of all ages, and it scares the dickens out of us.

Why? Because we know how dangerous a melanoma can be. It's the type of skin cancer most likely to spread to other parts of the body. It can be fast, devastating, and deadly. And it's affecting more and more women every year.

We know the major cause of it, and we think that we may know why its incidence is increasing. While sun damage has been clearly linked to melanoma risk, the thinning ozone layer in our atmosphere may be at fault for allowing higher levels of ultraviolet rays to reach people.

Unfortunately, we're not adjusting our lifestyles to counteract the increased number of ultraviolet (UV) rays. "Sunbathing and getting a 'healthy tan' are still very popular," says Mary Knapp, a state climatologist in the weather data library at Kansas State University in Manhattan. "And the use of sunblocks can lull people into a false sense of security, resulting in longer periods of sun exposure." In addition, clothing styles— from below-the-knee dresses to miniskirts and tube tops—continue to let the sun shine in to a

dangerous degree. What's more, family vacations to visit highly reflective ski slopes or perpetually sunny seashores may expose our children to more sun at an earlier age than ever before.

But despite all the grim facts, the news about melanoma is actually very good. In its earliest stages, melanoma is one of the easiest cancers to prevent, spot, treat, and cure.

Risk Factors

Want to know your chances of getting melanoma? Take a look in a mirror. If you have blonde or red hair (naturally, that is), green or blue eyes (under those colored contact lenses), and a porcelain complexion sprinkled with freckles, your risk of developing melanoma is anywhere from 10 to 20 times higher than that of someone with dark or black skin.

Looks aside, melanoma, like many other types of cancer, also appears to be related to our genes. That is, if a family member—your sister, your father, or even an aunt or grandparent—has had melanoma, your risk of the disease goes up. Like-wise, if you have already had a bout of melanoma, your chances of battling the beast again are higher than if you'd never had the problem at all.

In addition to pale skin and a family or personal history, other factors put you at increased risk for the cancer as well.

- Poor ability to tan
- A history of sunburns
- The presence of many (more than 50) normal moles
- The presence of unusual-looking moles
- An immune system that has been suppressed by medication or illness
- Excessive recreational or work-related sun exposure

Prevention

Is melanoma preventable? Yes, it's easy to prevent it: Stay out of the sun.

It's easy, that is, if you live and work in a cave. For the rest of us, who may enjoy spending an occasional day at the park, beach, or mountains, or even puttering in our own gardens, avoiding the sun is a little trickier. Here are some ways to help reduce your melanoma risk when you can't just avoid those rays.

Use sunscreen every day. Even in incredibly sunny climes, sunscreen works. "We can see this quite clearly in Australia," says Karen Burke, M.D., Ph.D., dermatologic surgeon at Cabrini Medical Center in New York City and author of *Great Skin for Life*. "Seventy-four percent of the population regularly uses sunscreen there. And their rates of melanoma are finally leveling off for the first time in decades."

But sunscreen is effective only if you choose it

BASAL CELL CARCINOMA

Melanoma may win the prize for most deadly skin cancer, but basal cell carcinoma is the most common. "It's actually the most common cancer in humans, period," says Tanya Humphreys, M.D., director of cutaneous surgery, laser surgery, and cosmetic dermatology in the department of dermatology at Thomas Jefferson University in Philadelphia. More than 800,000 basal cell carcinomas are diagnosed each year.

Basal cell carcinomas (BCCs) are *not* related to moles. Instead, they show up as pearly, translucent, or occasionally red-colored raised bumps, or nonhealing sores. BCCs typically occur on parts of the body that get intense, episodic sun exposure.

Most people who get basal cell skin cancers are over 40, but younger folks are not immune. Early childhood sun exposure may be responsible for the increase in basal cell carcinomas in young people, says Dr. Humphreys. "I've seen people in their late twenties and teens with this problem." Among those in their twenties and thirties, women seem to be more commonly affected, she says.

Basal cell cancers grow very slowly and rarely spread, but they can penetrate below the skin to the bone and do considerable damage where they lie. Surgery to remove the small tumors may leave little or no visible scarring, especially on the face. Some types of basal cell carcinoma are difficult to remove and may recur.

with care and use it properly. According to Dr. Burke, many dermatologists recommend sunscreen that has an SPF of at least 25 and is waterproof and capable of blocking UVA as well as UVB rays. Look for ingredients that physically block the sun, such as titanium dioxide and zinc dioxide. Sunscreens containing these large molecules actually form an invisible barrier on the skin and reflect the sun away.

Apply your sunscreen early, often, and with a heavy hand. Make your first application to all exposed skin at least 15 minutes before you plan to

SUSPECT MOLES: THE ABCs

Here are some warning signs that a mole or freckle should be seen by a doctor as soon as possible.

A

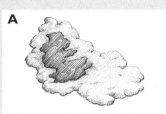

A is for Asymmetry: One side of the mole doesn't mirror the other.

B

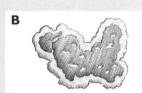

B is for Border: It should be smooth—not blurred, scalloped, or jagged.

C

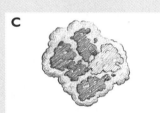

C is for Color: Color should be uniform, not varied. Black moles should be examined regardless.

D

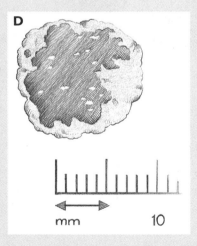

D is for Diameter: Melanomas are usually greater than 6 millimeters in diameter (larger than a pencil eraser).

mm   10

One more thing to watch out for: Some melanomas may be raised, like little hills. Any mole that begins to protrude from the skin should be examined promptly.

be outdoors. Then, reapply at least every 90 minutes, more often if you're swimming or sweating (okay, perspiring) a great deal, or possibly less often if you're using waterproof products. And be generous.

"When sunscreens are tested in the laboratory for effectiveness, an ample amount is applied per square inch. Most women apply much too thinly to get the amount of protection listed on the label," says Dr. Burke.

Check your skin regularly. Every woman knows about the importance of doing self-exams on her breasts. You can also give your skin a monthly once-over to look for changes in its appearance, particularly changes in moles or blemishes. Here's how, based on guidelines from the American Academy of Dermatology.

- Use a mirror to examine the front and back of your unclothed torso, including your arms and shoulders. Then, raise your arms and look at your right and left sides.
- Bend your elbows and look closely at your palms, forearms, and upper arms. Be sure to check both sides.
- Turn to look at the backs of your legs, then examine your feet, including the soles and the spaces between your toes.
- Use a hand mirror to help check the back of your neck in a wall mirror. Part your hair to examine your scalp.
- Last, use a hand mirror to look at your lower back and buttocks.

Go low-fat. Research shows that eating a low-fat diet may do more than just keep our hearts healthy and our weight steady. It may reduce our risk of skin cancer as well.

Thirty-eight people who followed a diet containing no more than 21 percent fat for 2 years slashed their average number of a certain type of precancerous skin lesion by as much as two-thirds when compared to people who ate a diet with no less than 36 percent of calories from fat, according to research at Baylor College of Medicine in Houston.

Following a low-fat diet in order to thwart your chances of developing skin cancer makes sense, says Shari Lieberman, Ph.D., a clinical nutritionist in New York City and coauthor of *The Real Vitamin and Mineral Book.* "After all, a low-fat diet has been shown to be protective against many other kinds of cancer," she says. "Why shouldn't it work for skin cancer, too?"

Signs and Symptoms

Malignant melanoma starts out as uncontrolled growth of pigment-making skin cells. The growth builds up to form dark-colored moles or tumors. They can appear on their own, on previously unmarked skin, but they can also, and often do, develop from or near an existing, formerly normal mole. This ability for healthy moles to become malignant is why learning the location and status of your normal moles through self-exam is so very important.

Any unusual change in your skin's condition should get your attention. New moles that appear on adult women are especially suspicious. That's

WOMEN ASK WHY

Why does drinking alcohol make my nose turn red?

If you find that every time you drink alcohol your nose gets red, you may want to start paying attention to your facial color at other times. You may notice that you tend to flush or blush after eating certain foods, like spicy dishes or things that come straight from the oven. You may also begin to realize that after vigorous exercise your face stays red far longer than anyone else's. One good way to really keep track of what's going on is to start a symptom diary: Record any flushing that you notice as well as when it happens and what you were doing, eating, or drinking just before it came on.

A predictable pattern of food, drink, or activity that triggers flushing may indicate that you have rosacea. Rosacea is a common skin problem that ranges in severity from persistent blushing and acnelike bumps to visible blood vessels and an enlarged nose. The condition happens much more frequently to women than men and can progress rapidly if not treated.

If you think that you may have rosacea, do yourself a favor and make an appointment to see a dermatologist. If you catch it early and treat it properly by avoiding triggers (including sunlight, a major cause of rosacea outbreaks for some people), you can keep the problem from getting worse.

Expert consulted
Lynn Drake, M.D.
Editor of Rosacea Review
Professor and chairperson of the department
*   of dermatology*
University of Oklahoma
Oklahoma City

because we've already developed most of the moles that we'll ever have by the time we reach adulthood. Be aware of any mole that begins to itch, bleed, ooze, or cause pain. Changes in size or shape should also alert you—moles shouldn't grow, and their edges should be smooth, not jagged. Research shows that color is particularly crucial in spotting melanomas. Be concerned

SQUAMOUS CELL CARCINOMA

Squamous cell carcinoma is the second most common nonmelanoma cancer of the skin. This threat is also sun-exposure-related, but rather than the one-time toasting that can cause melanoma, chronic long-term sunning seems to be the problem, says Tanya Humphreys, M.D., director of cutaneous surgery, laser surgery, and cosmetic dermatology in the department of dermatology at Thomas Jefferson University in Philadelphia. The cause is day-after-day unprotected exposure, such as farmers, mail carriers, gardeners, golfers, or runners get.

Squamous cell carcinomas often appear as raised red nodules or bumps or as red crusty or scaly patches. They often arise from precancerous lesions called actinic keratoses, which are extremely common, especially as we age.

Unlike melanoma, the chance that a squamous cell cancer will spread is small. But lesions on the relatively thin tissues of the lips or ears should be examined and removed promptly just to make sure that the cancer cells don't have the opportunity to travel.

about moles that are unevenly colored, with varied shades of brown and black. And if a mole suddenly turns color, especially to black, have your dermatologist check it immediately.

Don't Panic!

If you notice a new mole, don't automatically assume that it's a melanoma. The vast majority of moles are not dangerous, says Mary Gail Mercurio, M.D., assistant professor of dermatology at the University of Rochester in New York.

Even if you find a mole that has changed shape or has taken on a new hue, there's no need for immediate alarm (though a doctor's exam *is* in order). While the presence of abnormal moles, which are called dysplastic nevi, does mean that you may be at an increased risk for

melanoma, they don't all turn out to be cancerous. And, depending on your doctor's opinion, they may not even need to be removed.

Pregnancy can also make otherwise harmless moles darken. "That's not necessarily a bad sign," says Tanya Humphreys, M.D., director of cutaneous surgery, laser surgery, and cosmetic dermatology in the department of dermatology at Thomas Jefferson University in Philadelphia. "Estrogen can increase pigmentation." If you happen to notice a changing mole during pregnancy, bring it to a dermatologist's attention so that you can be monitored. But don't let it worry you unnecessarily.

Who Do I See?

Your own general practitioner or family doctor can certainly give you a routine screening for unusual spots or bumps during your yearly physical—be sure to ask if you'd like her to do so. But if you notice a new mole or a mole that's changing, you really should seek out a dermatologist, a medical doctor who specializes in the care and treatment of skin problems. "The key is in the diagnosis," says Lynn Drake, M.D., professor and chairperson of the department of dermatology at the University of Oklahoma in Oklahoma City. "Many doctors do things very well. But if you had a heart problem, you'd want a heart specialist. Likewise, with a questionable skin condition, it's best to see a skin specialist."

And don't delay. If there is a problem, early treatment is best for any skin cancer. And if it turns out that nothing is wrong after all, you will have saved yourself a lot of drawn-out worrying.

If you are diagnosed with a superficial melanoma, your dermatologist may be able to take it from there by removing the lesion herself. "Dermatologists are also wonderful surgeons," says Dr. Drake. But if the melanoma is deep, a medical-team approach might be warranted. In this case, your dermatologist may choose to partner with a surgical oncologist or other specialists who can give you the best treatment possible.

What Can I Expect?

After surgery to remove a mole, you may wind up with a visible scar. But the mark that removal leaves won't necessarily be as big as you are imagining right now. "The earlier you have something removed—that is, the smaller the mole is when it's taken out—the less severe your scar will be," says Dr. Drake.

After you have been diagnosed, have been treated, and have even physically healed, you may still feel the effects of melanoma somewhere else—in your mind. Suddenly, every freckle will seem fearsome. It's natural to react this way to a brush with what is, after all, a dangerous form of cancer. "Everyone who's had a cancer of any kind becomes a little more vigilant. It's a very scary experience," says Dr. Drake.

But it helps to realize that with melanoma, we really are lucky. With regular self-exams, we can catch it early. And with prompt treatment, the majority of women with melanoma will be able to get on with their lives—sunscreen bottle in hand.

Conventional Wisdom

The most important treatment for any new or changing mole is to have it examined right away.

MY MAMA TOLD ME
Will touching a toad really give me warts?

Quite simply, the answer is no. Touching a toad—or a frog, for that matter—may give you the willies, but never warts.

This old wives' tale probably got started because toads have warty-looking skin. Scientifically, however, the bumps you see on a toad's body are actually glands. If a toad feels threatened or in danger, these externally visible glands produce toxins that help the toad escape predators in ingenious ways. For example, if your dog picked up a toad in her mouth, the nasty-tasting toxins she'd taste would make her drool in response and drop the toad in the process.

We know that warts are produced by a specific type of virus that affects humans, and there's absolutely nothing like that located on a toad's bumpy skin.

Expert consulted
Lynnette Sievert, Ph.D.
Associate professor in the division of biological sciences
Emporia State University
Emporia, Kansas

Many dermatologists will use a specialized microscope to look closely at the mole and the surrounding skin. But in most cases, your doctor's trained eye is all that's needed to decide on the steps to take. "If a mole or other spot looks abnormal to my naked eye, I would proceed with a biopsy," says Dr. Mercurio.

Small questionable moles may be completely removed during the biopsy, and your doctor can perform this minor surgery right in her office. But if a mole is large or in an area where scarring is a concern, such as the face, she may decide to take a modest sample of skin to test before going further. All biopsied material is then sent to a pathologist, a doctor trained in detecting disease in the body's tissues, for thorough testing.

WOMAN TO WOMAN

She Discovered Her Own Skin Cancer

At 36, Catherine Poole, a Glenmoore, Pennsylvania, health writer, noticed a birthmark on her leg that suddenly looked different and unusual. Because she did something about it, she's alive today to tell her story.

In January 1989, I had a miserable flu. I was caring for my 2-year-old daughter, an editorial deadline was looming, *and* I was 5 months pregnant. But with all that, I guess you could still say that I was lucky.

Had I not been resting on the couch, I wouldn't have noticed the strange mark on the back of my calf. What had once been just a small birthmark now was bigger, black, and irregular in shape.

Because of its odd shape, I rushed to the dermatologist. A biopsy confirmed that I had a risky vertical-growth melanoma. Instead of spreading over the skin's surface, the cancer was burrowing deeper into the tissue. I had an 80 percent chance of living 8 years.

I was gripped with fear. Would I lose my baby? Would my kids lose their mom?

Doctors removed the cancer surgically and patched the area with a skin graft from my hip. It was a grueling and painful ordeal. I hobbled on crutches for the rest of my pregnancy. But I didn't care. They could take my whole leg as long as my kids had a mom.

After the surgery and the birth of my healthy son, I busied myself with research and realized that I'm in the high-risk category for this type of cancer.

I now consider myself a skin-cancer-prevention advocate. I'll tell complete strangers to have suspicious-looking moles checked. My doctor and I wrote a book called *Melanoma: Prevention, Detection, and Treatment* to help others recognize melanoma. And I helped establish the Foundation for Melanoma Research in Philadelphia to provide funding for research.

Needless to say, the experience changed my attitude toward the sun. Now, I always use sunscreen on myself and my family. And I get my skin checked regularly by my doctor.

If test results show melanoma and the entire mole was already removed at biopsy, you may have no further treatment to deal with. Superficial, or shallow, melanomas have the best chance of being dealt with this way. "Removal is the key with melanoma," says Dr. Mercurio. "Often, the surgery can cure the problem as simply as that."

Otherwise, surgery to remove the entire melanoma and a "safety margin" of surrounding skin will be in order. If your melanoma was elevated or had vertical growth extending into the underlying flesh, your doctor will want to carefully examine the rest of your body, especially your lymph nodes, to be sure that the cancer hasn't spread beyond your skin.

Chemotherapy drugs that are commonly used in treating other types of cancer aren't usually useful against melanoma. But therapy using a special protein called interferon has been successfully used to help some people with cases of melanoma that have spread.

Great Alternatives

When it comes to treating an existing melanoma, conventional Western medicine remains the proven best approach. But there are new and interesting tactics developing on the front lines that may become standard treatment in the future.

Keep an eye on the vaccine. New melanoma vaccines appear to have lifesaving potential. Custom-made for each patient from a sample of her own skin cancer cells, the vaccine augments her own immune system's ability to fight the cancer. Ongoing trials are only examining use in very advanced melanoma. And although the vaccine looks very promising, says Dr. Humphreys, there's still a long way to go.

Ask your doctor about B₆. A certain vitamin may also play a role in treating skin cancer. According to Dr. Lieberman, vitamin B_6 shows promise in inhibiting the growth of malignant melanoma cells. There are many other benefits for women who get enough of this B vitamin, including anemia prevention, better immune function, and possibly reduced PMS symptoms.

While the Daily Value for vitamin B_6 is only 2 milligrams, even that small amount is difficult to garner from food sources alone, says Dr. Lieberman. Some cancer specialists suggest that those at risk for melanoma as well as those being treated or who have had melanoma in the past take 100 to 300 milligrams of vitamin B_6 a day. This amount of B_6 should be taken along with a complete B-complex since B vitamins work synergistically, Dr. Lieberman adds.

But don't take this dosage without your doctor's approval. Excess vitamin B_6 can cause pain, numbness, and weakness in the limbs.

REAL-LIFE SCENARIO

She Thinks That Using Sunscreen Is More Dangerous Than Tanning

When Cindy goes to the beach, she goes prepared to protect her ivory-white skin. She wears a broad-brimmed hat, a terry-cloth robe, and wrap-around sunglasses. She also takes a beach umbrella. And she never leaves the house without slathering on sunscreen with an SPF of 20. Or at least she didn't until recently, when Cindy heard a news story claiming that sunscreen does more harm than good—that using it may actually promote cancer. Now she's confused. She loves the beach, but if she can't venture out from under her umbrella feeling secure that her skin is protected, she feels she may as well stay home. Should she?

If there's one thing Cindy *should* do, it's continue to use sunscreen. The controversy over whether or not sunscreens can actually increase the risk of skin cancer came about because of a presentation of misunderstood data that happened to catch the public eye. That said, there are a few reasons why it might be tempting to mistakenly think that sunscreen use leads to skin cancer, even though it probably does not.

For starters, people who use sunscreen the most religiously, usually very fair-skinned people who know that they burn easily, are also the ones genetically most likely to develop skin cancer in the first place. Next, once someone puts on sunscreen, she may tend to feel safe in the sun and stay out longer than she should. Finally, when people do use sunscreen, not many use it correctly.

Cindy is right to wear a hat and use an umbrella—these are great ways to protect herself from the sun whenever she's outdoors. But she would be even better off going one step further by using, every day, sunscreen with an SPF of 25 that protects against both UVA and UVB.

Expert consulted
Karen Burke, M.D., Ph.D.
Dermatologic surgeon
Cabrini Medical Center
New York City
Author of Great Skin for Life

Halt the Attacks on Womanhood: Reproductive Health

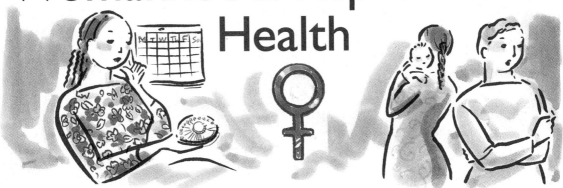

Serious illness is always worrisome, but it's especially so when it involves a woman's reproductive system. "Many women see their wombs as being tied up in who they are as females," says Yvonne Thornton, M.D., clinical professor of obstetrics and gynecology at the University of Medicine and Dentistry of New Jersey in Morristown and author of *Woman to Woman.* And since an estimated 37,400 cases of endometrial cancer and 25,200 cases of ovarian cancer are expected to be diagnosed this year, the worry is warranted.

Risk Factors

Simply being a woman puts you at risk for cancers of the reproductive organs. But there are other factors that can up the ante.

Age. Most ovarian cancers occur in post-menopausal women, half of them appearing after age 65. So your risk increases with each year, says Dr. Thornton.

Fertility drugs. "There may be a link between superovulation—the acceleration of ovulation that is usually the result of fertility drugs—and ovarian cancer," says Dr. Thornton.

A small family tree. If you had one or no children or you started your family later in life, you may be more likely to get ovarian cancer, says Joanna Cain, M.D., professor and chairperson of the department of obstetrics and gynecology at Hershey Medical Center of Pennsylvania State University in Hershey.

Family history. Has your mother, sister, or daughter been diagnosed with ovarian cancer? If so, you have an increased risk. Dr. Cain says that 5 to 10 percent of women whose close female relatives had ovarian cancer will also get the disease.

Obesity. A woman who is 30 pounds overweight has a tripled risk for endometrial cancer, and 50 extra pounds increases her risk tenfold.

Estrogen sans progesterone. When it's not coupled with progesterone, estrogen-replacement therapy increases your chances of developing endometrial cancer, says Dr. Cain. Taking the two together, however, actually decreases your risk. If you are taking estrogen and you experience bleeding or an abnormal discharge, see your doctor right away.

Talcum powder. If you've been exposed to talc—which was sometimes contaminated with asbestos until that was banned 20 years ago—either from direct application or from sanitary pads, your chances of developing ovarian cancer may be higher because talc may have a carcinogenic effect on the ovaries.

Prevention

Although oral contraceptives have long been maligned for *causing* cancer, they have actually proved to have a protective effect against hormone-related cancers that affect the uterus or ovaries, says Dr. Thornton. Birth control pills keep you from ovulating, so you're less likely to experience a cancer-causing malfunction, explains Lisa Domagalski, M.D., a gynecologist and assistant clinical professor at Brown University School of Medicine in Providence, Rhode Island. The Pill also ensures that you'll have a regular period each month, and the action of shedding the endometrium every 4 weeks makes conditions in your uterus less cancer-friendly.

"You don't have to take the Pill for long to enjoy its effects," adds Dr. Thornton. "If you take the pill from ages 20 to 21, you will still be reaping the protective benefits when you are 50."

If for some reason you can't take birth control pills—say you're a smoker or you have a history of migraine headaches—there are other ways to reduce your risk of ovarian cancer, says Beth Karlan, M.D., director of the Gilda Radner Ovarian Cancer Detection Program at the Cedars-Sinai Medical Center in Los Angeles. If you don't want to have any more children, you may have a procedure called tubal ligation, in which your tubes are tied, resulting in sterility. "Research shows that it can reduce your risk of ovarian cancer by up to two-thirds. The mechanism is unclear. One possible reason is that tubal ligation may inhibit the upflow of carcinogens into the abdomen," she explains.

Here are some other tips for prevention.

Get to the gynecologist. "Cancer can strike at any time, like lightning," says Dr. Thornton, "so it's important to screen for it with an annual pelvic exam." Even if you've had your children and gone through menopause, you need to get an annual gynecologic checkup.

OVARIAN CYSTS

The first thing to know about ovarian cysts is that they are actually part of what an ovary does normally. "Forming a cyst is often one of the normal consequences of ovulation," says Laurie Swaim, M.D., an obstetrician/gynecologist at Houston Women's Care Associates in Texas.

Cysts are just fluid-filled structures. They generally form and fade away during the menstrual cycle as a matter of course. Problems arise only when a cyst ruptures or grows too fast. And even when a cyst ruptures, the fluid is usually reabsorbed by the body with no further complications. "As a precaution, we might decide to observe the woman in the hospital for 24 hours," Dr. Swaim says, "but that's often the extent of it."

Of course, sometimes a cyst is more than just a cyst. While the presence of an ovarian cyst in a young woman is rarely cause for concern, the older a woman gets, the more worrisome any cyst becomes. That's because the risk for ovarian cancer rises with age. "You don't play around with a cyst in a woman over 35 or so. That's when an ultrasound is in order," says Dr. Swaim.

Ask for a CA-125 test. If you have other signs of ovarian cancer, blood tests can be done to screen for CA-125, a tumor marker that may indicate the presence of ovarian cancer in the beginning stages. "If I'd had this test as part of my annual exam, my cancer would have been caught before it spread throughout my entire pelvis," says Charlene Lynn, 58, a nurse in Houston, who was diagnosed in April 1998. Researchers at the Massachusetts General Hospital in Boston have concluded that regular CA-125 testing could save up to 5,000 lives each year. "I will yell from the top of the roof, 'Get a CA-125!'" says Lynn.

Watch your weight. Methods of preventing endometrial cancer are a bit more difficult to pinpoint. "Since we don't know what causes it, keeping in the best health you can is the best advice I can give," says Dr. Thornton. For one thing, that means staying slim—because a large number of women with endometrial cancer are overweight. Excess fat equals excess estrogen, and high estrogen levels put you at risk for both endometrial and ovarian cancer, she explains.

Eat whole foods. Another way to fend off endometrial cancer is to eat unprocessed fruits and vegetables, whole grains, and foods containing omega-3 fatty acids, recommends Katrina Claghorn, R.D., an oncology dietitian for the University of Pennsylvania Medical Center in Philadelphia. These whole foods may help boost your immune system and fight off reproductive cancers. "There seems to be a correlation between a high-fat diet and ovarian and endometrial cancers," she adds. So try to keep

your binges on ice cream and french fries to a minimum.

Signs and Symptoms

The number one symptom of endometrial cancer is abnormal—meaning, unscheduled—bleeding. That makes this type of cancer blessedly easy to detect, says Laurie Swaim, M.D., an obstetrician/gynecologist at Houston

ENDOMETRIOSIS

Endometriosis could be called the case of the wandering womb. For 10 percent of women between ages 25 and 50, endometriosis causes patches of uterine (or *endometrial*) tissue to migrate to locations outside the uterus. Strange as it sounds, these misplaced bits of womb, called endometrial implants, respond normally to female hormones, regardless of their location. When it's time for menstrual bleeding to occur, the implanted tissues begin to bleed as well.

Blood seeping from implants gets absorbed by other organs in the area—the ovaries, rectum, bladder, appendix, or even the lungs. This leads to irritation and the development of adhesions, dense internal scar tissue that can eventually build up to connect one organ with another. Severe menstrual cramps are the most common symptom, but pelvic pain, painful intercourse, and infertility—alone or in combination with each other—can also signal endometriosis.

Unfortunately, since the troublemaking bits of endometrial tissue are scattered within the abdominal cavity—and because symptoms associated with endometriosis could actually be signs of other problems—a surgical procedure called a laparoscopy is what's necessary to make an accurate diagnosis.

But before they do diagnostic surgery, most gynecologists would recommend that you try medications for 3 to 4 months, says Laurie Swaim, M.D., an obstetrician/gynecologist at Houston Women's Care Associates in Texas. "Since any surgery carries risks, we would rule out other possible causes, like infection or sexually transmitted diseases, then assume it's endometriosis and treat it medically."

As treatment for endometriosis, doctors often recommend contraceptive pills taken either continuously, to stop menstruation altogether, or as they would be for birth control, to help lighten menstrual flow and lessen the chance of backup. Synthetic hormones such as danazol (Danocrine) or leuprolide (Lupron) have also been used to treat severe endometriosis. While they can help relieve pain, both of these drugs have potentially problematic side effects, ranging from weight gain and deepening of the voice to hot flashes, depression, and osteoporosis.

Surgery can also constitute treatment for endometriosis. Adhesions or implants can be removed, cauterized (burned), or vaporized with a laser during laparoscopy, a procedure sometimes called belly button surgery because the small primary incision is made near the navel. In some cases, though, implants are too large or the organs involved are too delicate for laparoscopy, so *laparotomy*, or abdominal surgery, is the procedure of choice.

When endometriosis doesn't respond to medication or conservative surgery or when implants or adhesions recur, hysterectomy (removal of the uterus and ovaries) is an option. Women who have experienced crippling pelvic pain for years may find that this drastic-sounding measure brings the best and most reliable relief.

Women's Care Associates in Texas. Bleeding between periods isn't normal and should be checked out. "And postmenopausal bleeding of any kind needs to be investigated right away," she says. Even seemingly simple spotting should be brought to the attention of your gynecologist.

"Endometrial cancer can occur before menopause as well," says Dr. Cain. If you're bleeding heavily between periods, have continued heavy periods, or experience a very foul-smelling discharge, see your doctor, she adds.

Ovarian cancer, on the other hand, is quite a bit more difficult to discover. "Women aren't usually diagnosed until their cases are very advanced," says Dr. Swaim.

The problem is that there is no specific list of symptoms associated exclusively with ovarian cancer. Symptoms mimic everyday womanly complaints—cramping, bloating, abdominal swelling. "We cope and continue," says Dr. Karlan.

"I experienced some early-morning nausea and a slight change in my bowel habits, but I was going through a divorce, so I blamed it on my emotions," recalls Lynn.

"We need to begin finding ovarian cancer when it's in stage one—where cures can be effected most successfully," says Dr. Karlan.

There are ways to distinguish normal discomfort from the kind that should take you to your gynecologist. Troubling symptoms are constant, daily, and progressive, says Dr. Karlan. Pelvic pressure, bloating, urinary frequency, and constipation or any other change in bowel habits that lingers for a month should get your attention. "You know your own body," she says. "If you notice that suddenly your clothes fit tightly around your middle, have someone examine you."

Don't Panic!

The unexpected bleeding that can be a sign of endometrial cancer can also be a symptom of many other female complaints, ranging from the mild to the more serious. If you are premenopausal, you could have a polyp, a cervical infection, or fibroids, says Dr. Swaim. Don't let fear stop you from seeing your doctor.

Postmenopausal women do have more reason to worry about unscheduled bleeding. But even so, something harmless and correctable, like skipped or changed hormone-replacement medication, can often be to blame for spotting. "It's easy to test for endometrial cancer," Dr. Swaim assures. So get it checked out.

Symptoms that could mean ovarian cancer could also mean a host of other, non-life-threatening problems. Abdominal swelling could indicate fibroids, pregnancy, or a benign pelvic mass. Cramping or one-sided abdominal pain could be caused by a cyst or irritable bowel disease. Urinary frequency could be due to a bladder or urinary tract infection. Before you panic, see your doctor, then get treatment for whatever it is that ails you.

Who Do I See?

Any unusual bleeding should be evaluated first by your regular gynecologist. "As general gynecologists, we can treat most endometrial cancers," says Dr. Domagalski. If your case is more severe, you will most likely be referred to a gynecologic oncologist, a gynecologist specially trained in surgery and cancers of the female reproductive tract.

And be sure to ask if the doctor is board-certified, recommends Dr. Thornton. Certification

FIBROIDS

The slow-growing tumors commonly known as fibroids get called by the wrong name more often than not. The correct term for these common growths is *myomas*—the root of that word relating to muscle, specifically the uterine muscle where these tumors appear.

Fibroids seem to develop without any particular inspiration: Their cause, other than the simple presence of the female hormone estrogen, is somewhat of a mystery. A study conducted at the Mario Negri Institute of Pharmacological Research in Milan showed that women who frequently consume beef have 1.7 times the risk of fibroids. Eating a lot of fish, on the other hand, *lowers* a woman's risk by 30 percent.

The incidence is overwhelmingly common: One-fourth of all women have fibroids, with that rate rising to one-half in black women. While that sounds like a lot of women with "female problems," the fact is that the vast majority of fibroids keep to themselves, never causing the slightest complaint.

"So many women have them and don't even know it, because in so many women fibroids just aren't an issue," says Karen Meyer, N.P., L.M.W., a nurse practitioner and licensed midwife at the Pacific Fertility Center in San Francisco. Most

means your doctor has chosen to take national standardized oral and written tests in her field and can use the initials F.A.C. (for Fellow of the American College of the particular specialty). For example, F.A.C.O.G. stands for Fellow of the American College of Obstetricians and Gynecologists.

If your gynecologist decides that your symptoms suggest ovarian cancer, it's important that you choose a specialized doctor even *before* diagnostic surgery, says Dr. Karlan. "You want to have a gynecologic oncologist present at the initial surgery. It is very impor-

fibroids exist quietly during a woman's later reproductive life (they are most common around age 40) and then shrink away as estrogen levels drop at the time of menopause. Mild cases of fibroids may require no treatment other than close monitoring (of size and discomfort levels, for example) by you and your gynecologist.

Unfortunately, not all fibroids are silent. When fibroids grow large or multiply, they cause symptoms that are hard to miss and usually require medical treatment. Pressure on internal organs can lead to chronic pelvic pain. Fibroids can change the shape of your endometrium (uterine lining), often causing menstrual irregularities and frequent or extremely heavy periods, says Meyer. Other obvious indications that you may have fibroids are abdominal swelling, pain during intercourse, and urinary frequency or constipation.

Surgery is the most reliable way to end the heavy bleeding and possible anemia that come with large or multiple fibroids. For younger women who want to bear children, a procedure called myomectomy can remove the fibroids without removing the entire uterus. This type of abdominal surgery is complicated, however, and the growths do have a chance of recurring. If a woman with fibroids is already finished building her family, hysterectomy can be a sensible option that brings welcome relief.

What Can I Expect?

If you see your gynecologist because of unusual bleeding, she will most likely order an endometrial biopsy, which sounds worse than it is. She'll perform the procedure in her office. She'll use a thin catheter to retrieve a sample of endometrial tissue from the inside of your uterus. "You'll feel one giant menstrual-type cramp, and then it will all be over," says Dr. Swaim. No local anesthesia is used because there is no way that a doctor can numb your uterus, she says, and the procedure is so quick that general anesthesia is unnecessary.

If the test results reveal endometrial cancer, you will need surgery to "stage" the disease—that is, to discover how involved the cancer is and to determine the best course of treatment. Along with abdominal surgery to examine your uterus, your surgeon will probably want to biopsy some nearby lymph nodes as well. Further surgery, perhaps to remove your uterus, and chemotherapy may also play a part in your treatment.

tant that all visible tumor be removed the first time."

In addition to an M.D., you may choose to see a psychologist or a social worker to deal with the stresses you are facing pending or after a diagnosis of reproductive cancer, says Dr. Cain. "Because your entire family will be affected, I also suggest that you all attend counseling or group therapy together," she says. And an R.D. can help you with nutritional support. To promote general wellness, you may want to consult a naturopathic physician.

A suspicion of ovarian cancer will most likely lead directly to a trip to the operating room. There, a gynecologic oncologist will remove the mass and send it to a pathologist. If they think it is an early cancer, the surgeon will also remove one ovary, nearby lymph nodes, and tissue from neighboring organs to screen for cancer cells that may have spread.

A diagnosis of cancer of the reproductive organs presents emotional on top of physical challenges. "Women often think, 'I won't have a life without my uterus,'" says Dr. Thornton.

"Because of what women have learned about Gilda Radner's death, a suspicion of ovarian cancer will elicit a greater emotional response than endometrial cancer," says Dr. Domagalski. Radner, a comedienne of *Saturday Night Live* fame, died of ovarian cancer in 1989 at the age of 42.

"But when a woman is diagnosed with endometrial cancer, she may still assume the worst," says Dr. Domagalski. "Once she discovers how curable it is, she feels a sense of relief. With both endometrial and ovarian cancer, women just want it over with as soon as possible."

Conventional Wisdom

Most endometrial cancer is caught fairly early and surgically treated with hysterectomy, explains Dr. Domagalski. If the cancer is more advanced, the doctor may also decide to remove the ovaries, the fallopian tubes, the upper part of the vagina, or nearby lymph nodes. Sometimes, a period of radiation treatments, hormone therapy, or chemotherapy will follow.

The primary treatment for ovarian cancer is the surgical removal of the tumor, says Dr. Cain. If the case is more severe, one or both ovaries, nearby organs, and lymph nodes will be removed as well. Unfortunately, many cases of ovarian cancer are not cured by surgery alone, so chemotherapy is usually prescribed.

Great Alternatives

If you've been diagnosed with a cancer of the reproductive system or you want to reduce your

REAL-LIFE SCENARIO

Her Unusual Bleeding May Be More Than a "Heavy" Month

Four months ago, Rose, 39, started having unusually heavy menstrual periods. She thought nothing of it at the time, but the same thing has happened every month since then. She has also been bruising more easily, and her gums have started to bleed. When she mentioned her symptoms to a friend who is a nurse, her friend suggested she see a doctor right away. In the same breath, the friend rattled off the names of several life-threatening diseases, such as leukemia and aplastic anemia. Rose wasted no time. She went straight to her family doctor, who passed her directly to a hematologist. But after blood work had been done, the doctor tried to calm her. She had something called von Willebrand's disease—nothing to worry about. Well, she can't help herself. She's worried. Should she be?

The scenario above is a very common presentation for von Willebrand's disease. Although not everyone with this genetic abnormality has symptoms, often women with this problem experience nosebleeds, easy bruising, heavy menstrual flow, excessive or unusual bleeding from the mouth or gums, and occasionally, gastrointestinal or urinary tract bleeding.

chances of a future diagnosis, these alternative or complementary therapies may help boost your immune system.

Gulp some green tea. A number of studies performed in China and Japan indicate that people who regularly drink green tea have a lower incidence of cancer. The protective effects are thought to come from the antioxidants in the tea, says Helen Healy, N.D., a naturopathic physician and director of Wellspring Naturopathic Clinic in St. Paul, Minnesota.

Pop some selenium. The mineral selenium, which is found naturally in meat, dairy foods,

Von Willebrand's disease is the most common inherited bleeding disorder. It occurs when von Willebrand factor, a substance needed for clotting that's normally present in the blood, is lacking or abnormal.

Although it is a lifelong condition, von Willebrand's disease is easily manageable. Depending on the form of the disease (there are three types), treatment may consist of nasally administered desmopressin acetate (DDAVP) or a blood product called cryoprecipitate.

Any woman with symptoms that suggest von Willebrand's disease should be sure to get an accurate diagnosis—even if she has learned to live with the problem. That's because von Willebrand's is a genetic disorder, which means that if you don't know about it, you could unwittingly pass it down to any children you bear. Plus, any surgery, even simple elective ones, may require pretreatment with DDAVP to be safe.

Expert consulted
Deborah Goodman-Gruen, M.D., Ph.D.
Assistant adjunct professor of family and
preventive medicine
University of California
San Diego

and grains, has been shown to cut cancer risk by two-thirds. Selenium is most effective when taken in the supplement form, but be careful: taking too much can be toxic, warns Dr. Healy. Keep your daily dosage at 200 micrograms or less.

See yourself well. "Visualization helps you get in touch with the part of your body that is cancerous," says Dr. Healy. Also known as guided imagery, visualization uses the power of suggestion to create empowering images, such as a mass of cancer cells being attacked by the immune system.

Feed it back. Biofeedback helps you take an active role in your treatment. Through the placement of electrodes on your body and scalp, one of more than 10,000 biofeedback therapists in the country can teach you how to control some of your involuntary bodily functions, such as heart rate, blood pressure, and emotions. "Biofeedback is helpful for general wellness and chemotherapy-related nausea," says Dr. Cain.

Antioxidize. "For prevention of all types of cancer, taking antioxidants can be beneficial," says Claghorn. You can also get antioxidants from fruits and vegetables such as blueberries and red peppers. Stay away from antioxidants during radiation or chemotherapy, however, because they may reduce the effectiveness of the treatments.

Get some support. Psychological support is a necessary part of cancer treatment, Dr. Cain says. Information on cancer support groups is available at most hospitals.

Fight back. "I have no control over what this cancer is doing to me, but I have some control over what I'm doing to it," says Lynn. She has stayed in control of her illness by spreading the word to others. Thanks to Lynn's perseverance and some help from her daughter Nora, who works for the California Senate, a bill requiring insurance companies to cover testing for ovarian cancer is being negotiated. "I hope someone somewhere lives because my daughter loves me so much," Lynn says.

Shield Against Arrows to the Heart: Heart Health

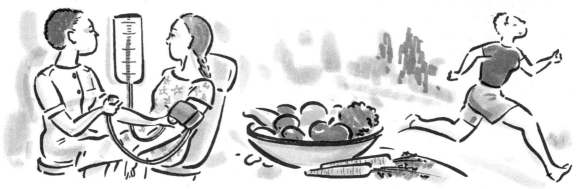

Most women consider breast cancer the greatest threat to their lives and health. But ironically, the greatest danger to our health doesn't lurk in the breast at all—it beats just beneath it.

For every woman killed by breast cancer, cardiovascular disease claims eight.

"Twice the number of women die of cardiac disease—heart attack, heart failure, stroke, all the cardiovascular diseases—as die of all cancers combined," says cardiologist Deborah J. Barbour, M.D., medical director of the coronary-care unit and director of the women's cardiovascular program at Mercy Medical Center in Baltimore. "People just don't know it."

We don't know it because we're used to thinking of heart disease as a male issue. "Our model for heart attacks is not a woman," says clinical psychologist Susan Brace, R.N., Ph.D., who practices in Los Angeles. It's the aggressive businessman keeling over, clutching his heart in the elevator and falling on his briefcase.

The truth is that heart disease is an equal-opportunity illness and has become the number one killer of American women. It appears when consistent exposure to the effects of stress, cou-

pled with high blood pressure, damages the inner lining of the arteries. A sticky blood fat called plaque then begins to accumulate on the damaged areas. Built-up plaque (atherosclerosis, or hardening of the arteries) narrows the arteries and invites blood clots, which reduce or even stop the bloodflow to the heart. The result can be a heart attack or a stroke.

Risk Factors

Heart disease and its awful sibling, stroke, are associated with several risk factors, as identified by the American Heart Association. You're stuck with some, but you can do a lot to change others.

First, here are the ones you can't change.

Age. Around menopause, your risk starts climbing and keeps going up.

Heredity. If a close relative has had heart disease or stroke, your chances of doing the same are increased.

Race. Black women are more likely to get heart disease and stroke than white women.

Health history. If you've had a heart attack or

stroke, you're at higher risk to experience either one at another time.

Here are the factors that you can do something about.

Smoking. Cigarettes skyrocket your risk. Even deadlier is the duo of smoking and birth control pills.

High blood cholesterol. A prime heart disease risk contributor, it is also a co-conspirator for stroke.

High blood pressure. Also known as hypertension, it's the biggest risk factor for stroke, and it's among the top 10 for heart disease.

Inactivity. You may think that a life of leisure is a dream come true, but your heart won't thank you for it.

Overweight. Too much fat, especially around the waist, can weigh you down with cardiovascular problems.

Diabetes. A woman with diabetes has up to seven times the risk of heart disease of one the same age without diabetes. But depending upon the type you have, diabetes can be controlled with insulin or with diet and exercise.

Stress. Though its role in cardiovascular disease isn't clear, unhealthy responses to stress, such as smoking and overeating, are recognized risk factors.

Prevention

Fortunately, if you have some of the changeable risk factors—and it doesn't matter how long you've had them—you can begin modifying and taming them immediately. Here are some places to start.

WOMEN ASK WHY

Why do you so often hear of men suddenly and without warning dropping dead of heart attacks, but you seldom hear the same about women?

This scenario describes a distinct health problem called sudden cardiac death (SCD). This isn't the "massive heart attack" that we hear about or even a heart attack at all. SCD can be caused by a heart attack, but often it is not. SCD is the result of cardiac arrest: The heart suddenly stops functioning because of a fatal change in the rhythm of its beating, and unexpected death occurs. The reason we don't hear about it striking women as much as men is that it's less common in women. Some researchers speculate that natural estrogen may help protect women against SCD.

In one study at Massachusetts General Hospital in Boston, researchers looked at underlying heart disease in male and female SCD victims. Women seemed less likely to have underlying coronary artery disease: 45 percent, compared to 80 percent for the men. So that suggests that women with coronary artery disease may actually be protected from SCD.

We need to find out how risk factors such as smoking, high blood pressure, and diabetes may differ between men and women. Prevention is key because the survival rate from sudden cardiac arrest is dismal—it ranges from 6 to 25 percent. Anything that can reduce risk is vital.

Expert consulted
Christine Albert, M.D.
Instructor in medicine at Harvard Medical
*   School*
Cardiac electrophysiologist at Massachusetts
*   General Hospital*

Snuff cigarettes. "Women smokers come to me asking about herbs and vitamins, and I say, 'Wait a minute,'" reports Sharonne N. Hayes, M.D., director of the Mayo Clinic

Women's Heart Clinic. "Your slightly elevated cholesterol's not going to kill you; your 10 pounds overweight won't kill you; but your smoking will." Gender is a minus here, says Dr. Hayes, because the same level of cigarette smoking puts women at greater risk of heart disease than men.

Get off that couch. Movement in the form of exercise tackles almost every preventable facet that underlies heart disease, says Elizabeth Ross, M.D., a cardiologist at Washington Hospital Center in Washington, D.C., and author of *Healing the Female Heart*. "It improves cardiac conditioning and lowers blood pressure, blood sugar, and stress. You couldn't ask for a better prescription."

This menu of heart-healthy benefits is supported by almost 100 studies, which were analyzed recently by two university doctors, one from the University of Toronto and one from Boston University Medical Center. They found that physical activities, such as walking, swimming, and aerobics, help lower blood pressure and prevent the development of high blood pressure, reduce cholesterol levels in the blood, discourage blood clots, and improve blood vessel performance.

Be lighthearted. Exercise also plays a big role in controlling another risk factor: obesity. Maintaining a healthy weight helps avoid the heart-related complications of obesity, according to Dr. Ross. "People who are obese tend to have lower activity levels, elevated cholesterol, diabetes, and higher blood pressure," she says.

Know your numbers. Too much

HIGH BLOOD PRESSURE

You can probably rattle off your height and shoe size, but how about your blood pressure? This measure of how hard blood pushes against blood vessel walls could be a number that saves—or threatens—your life.

For an adult, high blood pressure (HBP), also called hypertension, means that your pressure is 140 over 90 (140/90) or higher. The first number represents systolic pressure, that is, how hard your blood pushes when your heart beats. The second number is your diastolic pressure, which is the measure of the force your blood exerts when your heart is at rest.

Elevated blood pressure, according to the American Heart Association, signals that your heart is working harder than normal to pump blood and oxygen to your organs and tissues. That extra load puts you in extra jeopardy for a host of problems, including hardening of the arteries, heart attacks, and strokes.

Called the silent killer because it has no warning signs, HBP also has no known cause in upward of 95 percent of cases. What we do know, though, is that it more frequently strikes African-Americans, women who take birth control pills, people with diabetes, and those who are obese.

Medications can help control HBP, but there's a better treatment. "Exercise is probably the strongest medicine we have to combat HBP and heart disease," says Janice Christensen, M.D., assistant professor of clinical medicine at the University of Arizona College of Medicine in Tucson. "Most of the drugs available decrease your cardiovascular risk by 20 to 40 percent, but study after study shows that even moderate exercise cuts your risk of heart problems by up to 50 percent." Here are her tips for better blood pressure control.

Move it. Keep weight and blood pressure down by getting up and moving. For women especially, physical inactivity invites higher risk. To keep yourself healthy, get some form of moderate-intensity exercise—such as brisk walking, swimming, or aerobics—for at least 30 minutes most days of the week.

Follow doctor's orders. If you're on a low-salt diet or HBP medication, stick to it; otherwise, pressure can rise.

Do your homework. Because blood pressure rises and falls hour to hour, day to day, home monitors are useful for tracking readings. "Home monitors help you find your average pressure over months and years," says Dr. Christensen. She recommends the commonly available aneroid version, with the familiar stethoscope, arm cuff, and dial gauge, or a digital monitor with an electronic screen display. Ask for a lesson from your doctor or nurse on how to properly use your home monitor. Blood pressure readings will be inaccurate if your cuff is the wrong size, so you should also ask for your doctor's advice on the best size for you. Have your doctor check your machine for initial accuracy, then again annually.

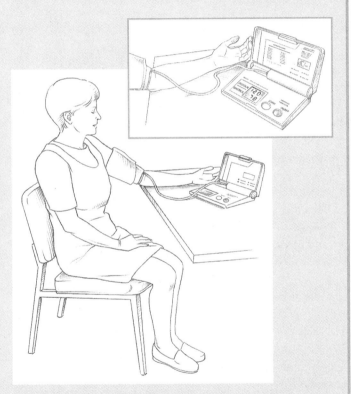

To use a home blood pressure monitor, sit with your back supported and your legs and ankles uncrossed. Place your arm at the level of your heart on a table or desk, and wrap the cuff around the upper part snugly. Some popular digital models will inflate automatically; for others, you will need to squeeze a rubber bulb. Your reading will appear on the display window or dial. Digital home blood pressure machines are portable and easy to use, with the controls and blood pressure readings clearly marked.

"bad," or low-density lipoprotein (LDL), cholesterol and high blood pressure hurt blood vessels and help heart disease advance, so it's important to keep your levels under control. Dr. Barbour's advice is basic and simple: Get your blood pressure and cholesterol checked every year. Your doctor will tell you how low they should be. And if you're on medication, don't stop taking it or make changes without checking with your doctor first.

Favor heart-smart foods. Your mouth helps determine heart health, too. For good nutrition, experts recommend that you emphasize fruits, vegetables, and whole-grain products, and eat fewer high-fat foods, such as baked goods, fried foods, chips, and packaged cookies.

Depressurize. To take some pressure off high blood pressure, experts suggest that you try one clove of garlic a day (stay away from the supplement form of garlic if you are on anticoagulants prior to surgery, because garlic thins the blood and may increase bleeding). They also suggest trying potassium (at least 3,500 milligrams daily from foods such as baked potatoes and cantaloupe) or a combined dose of 30 to 60 milligrams each of coenzyme Q_{10} and L-carnitine, sold in health food stores. Consult your doctor before taking L-carnitine, and keep in mind that coenzyme Q_{10} can cause a decrease in the effectiveness of the blood thinner warfarin (Coumadin).

Corral cholesterol. Experts offer a wide variety of nutritional options to control cholesterol. One of the newer herbal remedies is guggul, a resin from

STROKE

"Stroke" sounds ominous but vague. "Brain attack," though, zeroes in on the problem: the brain's supply of blood and oxygen is impaired, and brain cells can die. The symptoms, all sudden, include numbness or weakness of the face, arm, or leg, especially on one side; confusion; trouble speaking or understanding; trouble seeing in one or both eyes; dizziness; loss of balance or coordination; or extreme, unexplained headache.

Stroke is still the third leading cause of death, resulting in many more than 150,000 American deaths annually. It's also a chief culprit in adult disability in the United States. Two million Americans are estimated to struggle with the paralysis, loss of speech, and poor memory that stroke can bequeath, while one million bear little disabling evidence.

Sadly, women are the preferred targets of this cerebrovascular killer, constituting some 62 percent of stroke deaths. Those who smoke and take high-estrogen birth control pills are really in the crosshairs, bearing a stroke risk 22 times higher than average.

"Strokes are very common. People used to tell you that you couldn't do very much: Either you got better or you didn't," says Audrey S. Penn, M.D., deputy director of the National Institute of Neurological Disorders and Stroke in Bethesda, Maryland. "Today, though, prevention and acute treatment are really here."

Here is Dr. Penn's advice to help protect against stroke.

Manage high blood pressure. It's the biggest risk factor for stroke—and a key contributor to heart disease and kidney failure.

Stop smoking, period. Cigarette smoking promotes fatty buildups in your carotid arteries, the main highways for getting blood to your brain.

Get a heart checkup. Undiagnosed heart disease is a big threat since it can produce clots that cut down your brain's bloodflow.

Shake that body. "Exercise is good for everything—your heart, blood pressure, and helping to reduce your stroke risk," says Dr. Penn.

a tree grown in India. One study there showed a 24 percent drop in cholesterol after a 12-week regimen of 500 milligrams daily. Rarely, guggul may trigger diarrhea, restlessness, or hiccups.

Research also shows benefits from fenugreek, an herb available in seed or capsule form (1 to 2 tablespoons, or two 580-milligram capsules, taken three or four times daily), and a daily teaspoon of ground turmeric, the Indian herb you sprinkle on poultry, fish, and beans (or take a 150-milligram capsule of turmeric three times a day). Watch out for turmeric if you have high stomach acid, ulcers, gallstones, or bile duct obstruction.

Other cholesterol busters include a 3-ounce serving of fish with lots of omega-3 fatty acids, such as mackerel, salmon, and tuna; soy protein (pick your favorite soy product to get 47 grams per day); ground flaxseed (try a tablespoon on cereal, soup, or yogurt); and 500 to 1,000 milligrams daily of vitamin C.

Signs and Symptoms

While both sexes get cardiovascular disease, it's a mistake to assume that it can be diagnosed and treated the same way in each—a mistake that, by postponing care, could end up costing a woman her life.

Heart attack is the most visible sign of heart disease. It means that the vital supply of blood to the heart muscle has been reduced or halted and that immediate medical attention is urgent. "Women really don't have symptoms as clear-cut as men's," says Dr. Ross. While crushing chest pain is considered the classic red flag of heart attack, the warning signs for women may not wave as vividly.

You need to know when to act. Here's how.

Read the classics. The classic symptoms we most often associate with a heart attack include a feeling of pressure, fullness, squeezing, or pain in the center of the chest that lasts more than a few minutes; pain that spreads to the shoulders, neck, or arms; or chest discomfort accompanied by light-headedness, fainting, sweating, nausea, or shortness of breath.

Beware of *la différence*. Since women are more apt to have symptoms that aren't so classic or typical, according to Dr. Barbour, some other signs you should be aware of include breathlessness; tightness in the chest; sudden, overwhelming fatigue; and nausea.

Tightness or aching in the jaw, teeth, neck, throat, shoulder, or between the shoulder blades is also a warning sign.

Any one of these symptoms doesn't necessarily mean that you're having or about to have a heart attack, but it does mean that you should be checked out by your primary-care physician, advises Dr. Barbour.

Don't Panic!

Any heart attack warning sign may be due to a number of other conditions, some fairly minor.

GOING TO EXTREMES

Two diet and exercise plans that mandate extremely low levels of fat intake have documented success in lowering cholesterol and weight levels, but they require big lifestyle changes. Both plans, one created by Dean Ornish, M.D., and the other by Nathan Pritikin, call for limiting fat to as little as 10 percent of daily calories, exercising, and managing stress. Are they the answer for everyone? Probably not.

"For someone with a severe form of heart disease, the Ornish or Pritikin plan is probably okay," observes Beverly Yates, N.D., a naturopathic physician practicing in Seattle and author of *Heart Health for Black Women*. "But for the average person trying to be preventive, getting that fat intake down to about 10 percent is very tough."

"Ornish and Pritikin have done groundbreaking work," says Elizabeth Ross, M.D., a cardiologist at Washington Hospital Center in Washington, D.C., and author of *Healing the Female Heart*. "But you have to match the intervention with the severity of the disease—and the patient's ability to adapt." While she does recommend the strict low-fat regimens for some patients, Dr. Ross notes that many people are in too much of a hurry to comply with the programs.

Recently, four of the nation's top health organizations, including the American Heart Association, issued "Unified Dietary Guidelines" to help prevent heart disease and other killers. A ceiling of 30 percent of calories from fat is recommended, with the complex carbohydrates of fruits, vegetables, grains, and cereals pegged at a minimum of 55 percent.

"You don't need to see a cardiologist for every twinge," counsels Dr. Hayes. Sometimes, a feeling of pressure in your chest may be nothing more than a gassy souvenir of the bean dip you ate before dinner. But if your symptoms concern you at all, see your doctor.

Here are some other examples of conditions that can mimic a heart attack. Heartburn or esophageal reflux-type symptoms, where food and gastric juices flow backward from the stomach, can cause chest pain, says Dr. Hayes. She also notes that many joints, muscles, and their connections within the chest wall can be sources of discomfort.

And according to Dr. Barbour, chest symptoms can also be due to gallbladder disease, ulcers, panic attacks, or a variety of other causes.

Whether or not we have symptoms, many of us are actually more likely to brush off the threat of heart disease than to overreact, according to research. One study of 200 women ages 41 to 95 done at Stanford University School of Medicine found that only 34 percent knew that heart disease is the leading cause of death in older women.

Who Do I See?

For nonemergencies, the first stop is your family or primary-care physician. "If you have chest pressure, pain, nausea, or shortness of breath when you exercise, you should tell your doctor. These are all concerning symptoms," says Janice Christensen, M.D., assistant professor of clinical medicine at the University of Arizona College of Medicine in Tucson.

If a cardiac problem is suspected, you may be referred to a heart specialist, or cardiologist.

In alternative medicine, options abound—sometimes the same ones offered by conventional medicine. "Heart disease is an area where conventional and alternative medicine are beginning to merge," says Tori Hudson, N.D., a naturopathic physician, professor at the National College of Naturopathic Medicine, and

WOMAN TO WOMAN
Her "Silent Heart Attack" Finally Spoke Up

You can have a heart attack without even knowing it. Just ask Gladys M. Leist, 72, who didn't find out about hers until months afterward. Two more heart attacks later, the retired psychiatric nurse treasures her active, pain-free days. Here's her story.

My children and grandchildren all came to my house in Rochester, Minnesota, for a family dinner about 10 years ago. Right after we ate, I had a little pain in my chest, but I thought it was indigestion. I started feeling really rotten, so one of my daughters, who's a nurse, helped me to the bathroom. I passed out.

When I came to, I remember feeling really, really hot, so I asked my daughter to run some cool bathwater. When I got in the tub, I passed out again, so my daughter called the hospital emergency room. I felt okay after that, so I didn't go to the hospital and didn't really think much about it until I went for my yearly physical at the Mayo Clinic here a few months later. My doctor was looking over all the test results and said, "My gosh, Gladys, you had a heart attack, a silent heart attack. Did you know that?" I didn't.

My mother died of heart trouble when she was 62, so

director of A Woman's Time Clinic in Portland, Oregon.

"High-fiber, low-saturated-fat diets with lots of fruits and vegetables, eating soy, the importance of exercise . . . these are all things we naturopathic doctors have been practicing for years," she notes. "Now, clinical research backs us up." Not all heart disease can be treated effectively by a naturopathic physician alone, Dr. Hudson says. "If I have someone with dangerously high blood pressure, I'm calling up my nearest cardiologist and referring her for blood pressure medication before trying herbs and sup-

partly because of that I've always tried to take care of myself. I never smoked (except when I was 18, for maybe a year) always tried to eat right (lots of low-fat foods, fruits, and vegetables), and I exercise.

That's pretty much what the clinic doctor told me to do, and everything was fine for several years.

Then in 1994, on a visit to my daughter in Iowa, my heart spoke up loudly. On the morning I was planning to drive home to Minnesota, I got up feeling as if something were sitting on my chest. The pain didn't go away, but I still drove the 3½ hours back home. The pain just kept up, and I was sick to my stomach, too. Once I got home, I went to the emergency room at St. Mary's Hospital, where I had surgery called angioplasty to open up a blocked blood vessel.

Then things went pretty well again until last year, when I had another heart attack. I went to the Women's Heart Clinic at Mayo, and they implanted three stents. Those are stainless steel–mesh tubes that keep arteries open. Within a month, I was back to my full activities: I do aerobic exercises, I walk a lot, I use my treadmill at home, I garden, and I play ball with my two grandsons.

I'm not silent about heart disease; I talk to my women friends and family about risk factors, especially smoking, but a lot of them still smoke.

plements. Then, we'll see if we can gradually reduce her medication while integrating herbal and nutritional therapies."

What Can I Expect?

The physical aspects of cardiovascular disease take many forms, from heart attack to chronic chest pain, and so do the methods to diagnose it. In your doctor's office, a physical exam may start with the familiar cuff and pump to take your blood pressure. From there, depending on your risk factors, health history, and symptoms, you may have an electrocardiogram, a chest x-ray, an exercise stress test, or a nuclear imaging test.

Be wary of the exercise stress test, cautions Dr. Barbour. "Women tend to have false readings from a treadmill workout because women don't have the same response to exercise that men do." Instead, she prefers a stress echocardiogram or a stress test with imaging as a more reliable way to test the heart at rest and under exertion.

Emotionally, heart disease can have a frightful impact. "There's a 'terrified factor' with women who've had heart problems," says Dr. Brace. "They're really scared it might happen again."

A former coronary-care nurse who specializes in treating people with chronic and terminal illnesses, Dr. Brace sees a wide range of women's responses to heart attack. "Some women become more careful in a reasonable way, and some become what we call cardiac cripples: They're afraid to reach for the sugar because they might have another attack and die."

Some level of fear is perfectly normal, Dr. Brace relates, and so is grieving for a healthy heart. Medically, heart attacks are called MIs (myocardial infarctions). "The *infarction* means that part of the heart muscle didn't get blood and died," she says.

The grief response is extremely common in women diagnosed with heart disease, affirms Dorothea Lack, Ph.D., clinical assistant professor in the psychiatry department at the University of California, San Francisco. "There's guilt (thinking they caused the disease themselves by not exercising or eating healthfully), denial, shock, rage, depression, and, finally, acceptance."

Of course, different women handle their heart disease differently, reports Dr. Lack, who specializes in the psychology of medicine. Someone who handles life's challenges in a relaxed, accepting way is probably going to do better than someone who is anxious and driven. A litigation lawyer is not going to do as well as a yoga teacher, she observes.

Here's what the two psychologists find most effective in helping women handle heart disease.

Cry if you want to. Being upset is a normal part of serious illness. Try to accept your feelings.

Be helpless sometimes. "Women caretake other people so much that we think we're not supposed to get sick. There are some things we can't fix or change," says Dr. Brace.

Give yourself positive messages. "The thought process is a key part of rehabilitating a cardiac patient," Dr. Lack avows. People make their own 'audiotapes' that they play over and over in their minds. It's important that they find out what messages they're sending themselves and if they're negative, try to change them, she adds.

Conventional Wisdom

Today, there are reasons to be positive if you're diagnosed with heart disease, affirms Dr. Hayes. Conventional medicine offers several treatment options and procedures, some especially good news for women.

Diagnosis. A noninvasive test known as electron beam computed tomography (EBCT) can detect heart disease in women who have no out-

WOMEN ASK WHY

Why do they say that flossing my teeth can help my heart?

The connection is the bacteria in plaque, that invisible, sticky film that forms on your teeth. Without daily flossing, brushing, and periodic professional care to remove that plaque, you can develop periodontal (gum) disease, as do three out of four Americans over the age of 35. Gum disease bacteria can gain entry to your bloodstream through injured tissue. Ultimately, these bacteria can contribute to narrowed arteries and blood clots, which can lead to heart attacks.

Our research team at the University at Buffalo School of Dental Medicine was among the first to find a link between plaque bacteria and the risk of heart attack. During one of our studies, we found that people who had one of the more damaging types of oral bacteria had up to a 300 percent greater risk of heart attack than people without the bacteria. Continuing research lets us say with certainty that you cannot be healthy without oral health.

Here are the latest recommendations.

Get a physical for your mouth. At every regular dental checkup, don't just ask if you have cavities. Ask about your

ward symptoms. The EBCT rapidly scans the beating heart with x-rays in search of problems in the arteries.

Medicines. Taking drugs called statins may reduce a woman's cholesterol and will consequently reduce her chances of having a first heart attack, says Dr. Hayes. An aspirin a day can work as a preventive method for a woman who has already had a heart attack. Long-acting drugs called nitrates and beta-blockers can be taken for chronic chest pain.

Devices and materials. To open the arterial highway for better bloodflow to the heart, doc-

plaque accumulation; get a complete probing of your gums once a year.

Ask for flossing feedback. You can be diligent about flossing and not be effective at removing plaque if your technique or flossing material isn't right for you. Show your hygienist your flossing technique and discuss your brushing habits. Ask what you can change to improve your oral health.

Buy right for your mouth. With all the different toothpastes, aids, and flosses on the market, it's easy to be misled. Tartar-control toothpastes benefit some, not all, people; mouthwashes that have an antibacterial effect are available; some floss is coated to resist shredding. Your oral-care program shouldn't be built around advertising. Ask your hygienist and dentist what's best for you.

Like taking a shower and washing your hair, oral health used to be regarded merely as part of your daily routine. Now we know that the prevention of oral disease is far more important than we used to believe.

Expert consulted
Sara Grossi, D.D.S.
Clinical director
Periodontal Disease Research Center
State University of New York at Buffalo

tors can perform a balloon angioplasty, inserting a catheter or tube into a narrowed artery and literally inflating the balloon. To keep widened arteries from reclosing, doctors can implant a stent, a wire-mesh tube. And there have been huge advances in the catheters, metals, and computers used for these and other procedures, says Dr. Hayes. "Arteries that we wouldn't have touched 3 years ago we're doing successfully now. This is a particular advantage for women, because their arteries are smaller than men's."

Surgery. There's a less invasive type of bypass surgery where the incision is made under a breast, reports Dr. Hayes. And for people who are not eligible for a bypass because of certain obstacles, such as the locations of their blockages, one investigational technique seems to be promising. The new procedure involves using a laser beam to foster the growth of new blood vessel cells.

Great Alternatives

Alternative and conventional medicine are pretty much in sync on several key aspects of preventing and treating heart disease: exercise, nutrition, and stress management. "There's a huge variety of things alternative medicine can do here," attests Beverly Yates, N.D., a naturopathic physician practicing in Seattle and author of *Heart Health for Black Women.* Here are some preferred therapies.

Manage your minerals. If a woman is athletic or eats a poor-quality diet high in saturated fats and trans fatty acids, she may need extra magnesium and calcium, says Dr. Yates. Typical dosages are 350 milligrams a day of magnesium oxide and 1,200 to 1,500 milligrams daily of calcium carbonate. People with heart or kidney problems should check with their doctors before taking supplemental magnesium.

Eat your herbs. For women with high blood pressure or high cholesterol levels, Dr. Yates deploys a varying arsenal of herbs: hawthorn, shown to open arteries and improve bloodflow to the heart; ginkgo, for its dual action in strengthening vein tissues and enhancing brain bloodflow; and garlic, which has been shown to help decrease high cholesterol levels and increase "good" high-density lipoprotein (HDL) cholesterol. Dr. Yates also suggests trying citrus fruits and berries for their bioflavonoids, compounds that strengthen blood vessels.

Step up soy. Soy flour, soybeans, tofu, whatever the form, Dr. Hudson says to aim for 47 grams of soy protein a day. That was the average amount, she reports, in a summary of 38 clinical trials showing cholesterol reductions of more than 9 percent through soy protein intake.

Go high fiber. Yes, a bowl of oat bran cereal or oatmeal each day can help lower cholesterol levels by 8 to 23 percent in as little as 3 weeks, advises Dr. Hudson. These and other sources of soluble fiber, such as fresh fruits and beans, promote the intestines' ability to excrete cholesterol.

Downplay "bad" fats. Saturated fats, typically animal fats, are associated with higher cholesterol levels. Instead, Dr. Hudson urges, reach for monounsaturated oils, like olive and canola oils, and steer clear of margarine. "Margarine is an unsaturated fat that has been made into a saturated fat," she explains. "Margarine raises the bad LDL cholesterol levels, lowers the good HDL cholesterol, and can therefore increase the incidence of heart disease."

Find "good" fats. For the clot-busting, blood pressure–lowering benefits of omega-3 fatty acids, reach for salmon, tuna, halibut, mackerel, and herring, advises Dr. Hudson.

Fend Off Personal Attacks: Sexual Health

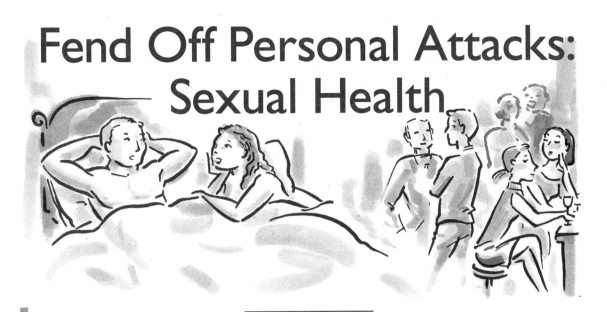

If you've made it past the age of 26 without contracting a sexually transmitted disease (STD), you've been either very lucky or very prudent. Nearly two-thirds of all cases in the United States occur in people who are younger than that. But no matter what your age, if you're still chasing after those wild oats and having unprotected sex—even with seemingly "nice" guys—your risk for getting an STD is as high as any 18-year-old's.

STDs are transmitted by close intimate contact—through sexual intercourse or oral sex. The organisms causing them are found in semen, vaginal secretions, saliva, or the skin around the genitals or mouth. These organisms can be of all sorts—bacteria, viruses, even protozoans, which are somewhat similar to the microscopic critters that live in pond water. All of them can invade your sexual organs, and most of them can also invade your mouth, throat, and anus. Some of these organisms, such as the corkscrew-shaped bacteria of syphilis or the tiny virus that causes AIDS, can spread throughout your entire body. And many can be transmitted to your baby if you have the infections while you're pregnant.

Risk Factors

The more sex partners you have, the more likely you are to pick up any kind of STD. But even if you have only one sex partner, if that partner has unprotected sex with others, you're still at increased risk. "I've seen women who didn't realize that their husbands were having affairs until they came down with STDs," says Shirley Glass, Ph.D., a psychologist practicing in Baltimore. In fact, there's evidence that men may be less safety-conscious about sexually transmitted diseases than women may like to believe. One study found that men who'd had a previous STD were almost three times more likely to engage in unprotected sex than men who had never had one. Women, on the other hand, were more likely to use protection if they'd had a previous infection.

Common vaginal infections such as trichomoniasis (which is itself an STD), bacterial vaginosis, and yeast vaginitis make you more likely to develop an STD if you're exposed to it. That's because these infections, minor as they may seem, disturb the natural defense mechanisms of

SYPHILIS

The English and Italians called it the French disease, the French called it the Italian disease, the Russians called it the Polish disease, and in Spain, where it was first recognized, it was called the disease of Haiti. We call it syphilis.

Syphilis starts with the appearance of a small, painless ulcer, called a chancre, on the spot where the bacteria entered your body. The chancre lasts for 1 to 5 weeks and then heals on its own. In the meantime, however, the bacteria spread throughout your body. Some time later, you may have a secondary outbreak in the form of lesions, swollen glands, hair and weight loss, slimy white patches in the mouth, muscle aches, and fever. It's possible to get syphilis just by touching someone who has these lesions. Eventually, the lesions go away, and about one-quarter of people appear to be healed. Another one-quarter have antibodies to syphilis but show no symptoms.

In the remaining half of the people with syphilis, the infection appears a third time, as long as 5 to 40 years after the initial infection, and can cause extensive brain damage, mental illness, and death. Good reason to get your penicillin within a year of your first exposure.

your vagina and cervix, so these infections should be treated promptly.

And if you have one STD, chances are higher that you also have a different one along with it.

Prevention

Despite impressive advances in treatment, prevention is still your best bet. And prevention can be summed up with one of two words: *abstinence* or *condoms*. Short of not having sex at all, condoms are the most effective method for preventing transmission of STDs, says Mary Lake Polan, M.D., Ph.D., professor and chairperson of the department of gynecology and obstetrics at Stanford University School of Medicine.

"The spermicide nonoxynol-9 has been said to be somewhat effective in the prevention of STDs, but it's not as good as condoms." Using a spermicide in combination with a latex condom may be more effective than condoms alone.

Remember, however, that although using a condom reduces your risk for STDs, it does not eliminate the risk entirely. You can still pick up infections orally or from areas of skin that are not covered. Male and female condoms work equally well at preventing most diseases, but the female condom has a slight advantage when it comes to preventing genital herpes and warts, since it keeps a bit of skin around the outside of the vagina from coming in contact with the penis.

As for other birth control devices, don't put your faith in them when it comes to preventing disease. "Diaphragms and cervical caps provide little or no protection and should not be used to prevent an STD," Dr. Polan says.

Some STDs can be knocked out with drugs, but others simply cannot. These include those caused by viruses: human papillomavirus, which causes genital warts; human immunodeficiency virus (HIV), which causes AIDS; herpes; and sexually transmitted forms of hepatitis (types B and C). Most of these viral infections persist in your body for the rest of your life, but that does not necessarily mean that you will be ill for life, says Anne Rachel Davis, M.D., assistant professor of obstetrics and gynecology at New York Presbyterian Hospital in New York City.

Health problems caused by STDs tend to be more severe and more frequent for women than for men because women often don't develop symptoms that cause them to seek treatment until the disease has gained a stronghold, Dr. Davis says. By that time, infection may have spread to the uterus and fallopian tubes and developed into pelvic inflammatory disease, a major cause of infertility and ectopic pregnancy (pregnancy in the fallopian tubes, which can be fatal if not diagnosed and treated promptly). And sometimes the symptoms of an STD are mistaken for a disease not transmitted through sexual contact. For instance, pelvic inflammatory disease, caused by chlamydia or gonorrhea, can be confused with endometriosis.

Some women mistakenly believe that if they simply get a Pap test each year, it will reveal if they have an STD, but that's a potentially harmful misunderstanding, says Amy Hughes, M.D., professor of obstetrics and gynecology at Medical College of Georgia in Augusta. It simply isn't true.

What's more, many women—and their gynecologists—follow a don't-ask, don't-tell policy. During an office visit, neither patient nor doctor brings up the subject of possible exposure to an STD. That, too, can cause serious problems down the road.

Signs and Symptoms

Symptoms vary according to which STD you have, but they often include vaginal discharge, odor, or itching, and may include pain or pressure. If you have herpes, you may develop blisters in and around your vagina and feel as if you have the flu. If you have genital warts, you'll develop painless, small, fleshy growths. If your infection develops into pelvic inflammatory disease, you'll have pain in your pelvic area and possibly a fever.

Don't Panic!

If you're experiencing symptoms, there's no need to immediately point a finger at a sexual partner. There are other possible explanations

---

GONORRHEA

An estimated 800,000 new cases of gonorrhea occur in the United States each year. The early symptoms are often mild, and many women who are infected have no symptoms at all. If symptoms do develop, they usually appear within 2 to 10 days after sexual contact with an infected partner, although some people may be infected for several months without showing any signs of the illness. Initial symptoms in women include a painful or burning sensation when urinating and a yellow or bloody vaginal discharge. More advanced symptoms indicate that the disease has progressed to pelvic inflammatory disease and include abdominal pain, bleeding between menstrual periods, vomiting, and fever. Men usually have more symptoms than women, with discharge from the penis and a burning sensation during urination that may be severe.

Gonorrhea can be diagnosed with several different tests. Doctors often choose to use more than one because results can be inaccurate. Because penicillin-resistant cases of gonorrhea are common, other antibiotics are sometimes used to treat the disease, most often ceftriaxone (Rocephin), which a doctor can inject in a single dose. Since gonorrhea can occur together with chlamydia, doctors usually prescribe a combination of antibiotics, such as ceftriaxone and doxycycline (Doxycin).

If you have gonorrhea, your sex partner should be treated as well, even if he has no other symptoms.

GENITAL HERPES

If you have genital herpes, join the crowd. About one in four U.S. adults have herpes, and as many as 500,000 new cases are thought to occur each year. Once you get herpes, it's forever. There's no cure for this viral infection.

Most people who are infected with herpes never develop symptoms. When symptoms do appear, they vary widely from case to case. The first symptoms usually appear within 2 to 10 days of exposure to the virus and last an average of 2 to 3 weeks. Early symptoms may include itching or burning; pain in the legs, buttocks, or genital area; vaginal discharge; or a feeling of pressure in the belly. Within a few days, small red bumps appear at the site of infection that may later develop into blisters or painful open sores. Over a period of days, the sores crust over, then heal without scarring. Some people also develop fever, headache, muscle aches, and swollen glands in the groin area.

There are two types of herpes viruses, genital and oral, but the oral type can also cause genital herpes, and genital herpes can infect the mouth.

Recurrences are more likely to happen if you're under stress, ill, or menstruating.

Herpes can be accurately diagnosed only by viral culture, which means that your doctor must take scrapings from your sores when they first appear. If you get tested after your sores are no longer active, the results may be negative even though you have the virus.

It's possible to infect someone with the virus even when you have no sores. That's because the virus can reactivate without causing sores. It's important to avoid direct contact with skin that contains the virus. Since recurrent outbreaks are not always apparent, you should always wear a condom if you or your partner is infected with the herpes virus.

Antiviral drugs such as acyclovir (Zovirax) can help people with a first or a recurrent outbreak of herpes. The medicine interferes with the virus's ability to reproduce.

for your discomfort. "Both urinary tract infections and yeast infections can mimic the symptoms of an STD," says Dr. Polan. These symptoms include painful urination, increased frequency of urination, and vaginal itching.

"Dermatological reactions to clothing or certain chemicals or perfumes can also cause problems similar to those of an STD, especially itching," adds Suzanne Trupin, M.D., clinical professor in the department of obstetrics and gynecology at the University of Illinois College of Medicine in Urbana-Champaign and coauthor of *Sexually Transmitted Diseases: Problems in Primary Care.*

But if you think that you may have contracted one of these infections, it's best to see your doctor to confirm the medical reason for your discomfort, especially if you have pelvic pain or a fever. "Many STDs have no symptoms, and that's really the biggest problem," says Dr. Polan. "With no symptoms, there's no way to know if you have an STD except for a culture, and cultures are often inaccurate. That's why prevention is so important. Although some STDs are difficult to diagnose, if they are caught early, many can be cured with today's modern antibiotics."

Who Do I See?

Gynecologists traditionally treat female STDs, but don't presume that if you have something, your doctor will find it on her own, Dr. Hughes says. Tell her about your symptoms or concerns so she can do the proper tests and examination.

What Can I Expect?

If you suspect that you have an STD, you may undergo a microscopic examination of your vaginal secretions, or you may have a culture to see what organisms are causing the problem. Some of these diseases require careful examination of the cervix with a lighted magnifying tube, a procedure called colposcopy. If you have reason to suspect that you've been exposed to HIV, you will need to have a blood test to look for antibodies to that disease.

If your tests confirm the presence of one of these illnesses, you will most likely feel a range of emotions in addition to the possible physical discomfort. If an STD takes you by surprise, you may feel enraged, violated, and betrayed—and perhaps angry with yourself for allowing yourself to be exposed to the illness. But no matter how angry you feel, take time to stop and think calmly about what has happened. "One important aspect of the emotional response is trying to determine how the STD was acquired in order to prevent a future occurrence," says Dr. Trupin.

If you're diagnosed with AIDS, you'll probably have much stronger feelings. "Most women feel the same sort of emotions as others with potentially terminal illnesses—hopelessness, grief, anger, and denial—but with the added social stigma that HIV carries," says Dr. Trupin. "The most common emotions that women with HIV/AIDS face are depression and anxiety."

GENITAL WARTS

Genital warts are flat lesions or small fleshy cauliflower-like bumps that can grow in and around your cervix, vagina, and anus, or, in men, on the penis and scrotum and in the urethra. The warts are usually painless, but they may itch. They are caused by the human papillomavirus (HPV). Several strains of the virus have been linked to cervical cancer, but these strains do not always produce visible warts. It's possible to have your warts analyzed to see which strains of virus you have.

You can get these growths through direct contact with someone else's warts, but the virus can also be spread through bodily fluids such as semen or vaginal secretions.

The warts are diagnosed by a doctor's visual examination and are removed by the use of chemicals, freezing, burning, or a laser. The warts return at least 30 percent of the time, however, so you may need more than one treatment.

Getting regular Pap tests can reveal the presence of precancerous or cancerous cells caused by HPV. A biopsy is warranted if the warts are brown or black, if they look unusual in some way, if they are larger than a thumbnail, if they are red and scaly, and—regardless of the nature of the warts—if a woman has an abnormal Pap test.

Some women even contemplate suicide, she adds. But an AIDS diagnosis is no longer a death sentence. In many cases, new medicines have helped slow HIV's progression to AIDS. "It may be very helpful to talk to women who have gone through the same problems," advises Dr. Trupin. "There are a number of national and local support groups that can be very useful in coping with different aspects of the disease."

Conventional Wisdom

Doctors use a whole arsenal of drugs and treatments to try to knock out STDs. The

HIV/AIDS

While just 7 percent of AIDS cases in 1985 were attributed to heterosexual sex, that number rose to 23 percent in 1998.

Of the infections among women, 75 percent are due to heterosexual sex and 25 percent to injection-drug use. Still, women account for only 30 percent of new infections. And of that percentage, Black women account for 64 percent, while Hispanic and White women account for 18 percent each.

A woman can contract HIV if her HIV-infected partner is an IV-drug user or bisexual or has been in the past. Two new studies suggest that bisexual risk behaviors among Black men may be fueling the spread of HIV infection to Black women in some parts of the country. One study, done in New York City, found 20 percent of Black men reporting bisexuality, compared to 4 percent of White men.

Women are also more vulnerable to getting HIV if they have some other sexually transmitted disease or if they have anal sex. It is also possible to contract HIV from oral sex.

Male-to-female transmission of the virus is eight times more efficient than female-to-male transmission, so men are much more likely to spread the virus to women than women are to men.

The average time between the initial infection and the appearance of symptoms that could lead to a diagnosis of AIDS is 8 to 11 years. This time varies greatly from person to person and depends on health status and behavior. Many people don't have any symptoms for many years or have mild symptoms of swollen lymph nodes and fever. Then, as AIDS develops, they experience weight loss, fatigue, diarrhea, and development of opportunistic infections that take advantage of their bodies' ravaged immune systems.

If you think that you're at risk for having HIV, get tested. Current tests for HIV are among the most accurate medical tests available.

If you test positive, you can take drugs that may downgrade HIV from a death sentence to a chronic disease, including AZT (Retrovir), also known as zidovudine or azidothymidine, and protease inhibitors like ritonavir (Norvir) and saquinavir mesylate (Invirase).

choice depends entirely on which STD you have and, sometimes, how long you've had it. For instance, if you've had syphilis for less than a year, it can be cured with one dose of penicillin. Those who have had it longer will need additional doses.

Women with genital herpes may take an antiviral drug, such as acyclovir (Zovirax), to lessen the severity of an initial outbreak or to reduce the number of recurrent outbreaks. Women with genital warts can have them removed with chemical-peel creams, laser surgery, freezing, or cauterization. Women with HIV infection can take a combination of antiviral drugs, usually zidovudine (AZT) and protease inhibitors. In some people, these help to stop the virus from multiplying.

In most cases, if you have an STD, so does your sexual partner. He needs to be treated for the same problem.

Great Alternatives

Once your infection has been brought under control, you can use alternative medicine to help maintain vaginal health and to rebuild your immune system, says Jody Noe, N.D., a naturopathic physician in Brattleboro, Vermont. Here's what she suggests.

Adopt a healthy diet to strengthen immunity. Our bodies' response to any infection depends on the ability of our immune systems to gear up to fight it, and that requires good nutrition. It's important to get adequate amounts of all the vitamins and minerals, especially vitamins A, C, E, and B complex, and the minerals zinc and selenium. It is also crucial to stay away from too much sugar and to balance adequate amounts of high-quality protein with carbohydrates. Whole grains, fish, beans, lots of vegetables, and fruit all fit this bill.

If you have a viral infection, consider trying N-acetylcysteine (NAC). This nutritional supplement, available in health food stores, may act as "a general antiviral," Dr. Noe says. She recommends that people who have AIDS or hepatitis B or C take 1,000 to 2,000 milligrams a day of NAC. People with recurrent herpes infections may also benefit from taking this amount. Check with your M.D. before taking cysteine. In high doses, cysteine can cause kidney stones in people who have cystinuria. Since it may inactivate insulin, use with caution if you have diabetes. Cysteine may also deplete zinc and copper, so if you're supplementing cysteine or N-acetylcysteine for more than a few weeks, take it with a multivitamin/mineral supplement that supplies the Daily Value of these minerals.

Don't douche unless your doctor recommends it. Studies show that women who

---

CHLAMYDIA

This sexually transmitted disease gets its name from the Greek word for "cloaked." And chlamydia, caused by the *Chlamydia trachomatis* organism, lives up to its name. Often, it initially has such mild symptoms that a woman does not know she is infected. If left untreated, the chlamydial infection may lead to pelvic inflammatory disease (PID). PID can result in scarring of the fallopian tubes, which can then block the tubes and make conception difficult or impossible. Often, men also have no apparent symptoms and can unknowingly pass the infection along to their partners.

Chlamydia can set up shop not only in your reproductive organs but also in your mouth, throat, eyes, anus, and lymph nodes.

The best way to diagnose chlamydia is for your doctor to get a sample of secretions from your genital area for laboratory analysis.

Chlamydia can be knocked out with antibiotics, often azithromycin (Zithromax) or doxycycline (Doxycin). Your sex partners must be treated, too. Penicillin (Robicillin VK), which is often used for treating some other sexually transmitted diseases, is not effective against this one.

---

douche are actually more likely to develop pelvic inflammatory disease than those who don't, perhaps because the process disrupts the balance of protective organisms in the vagina, allowing faster growth of unfriendly organisms. Instead of douching, see a doctor if you develop an unusual discharge or smell.

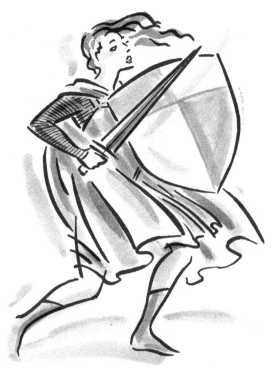

PART THREE

Holding
the Line

Unwelcome Occupiers: Chronic Illnesses

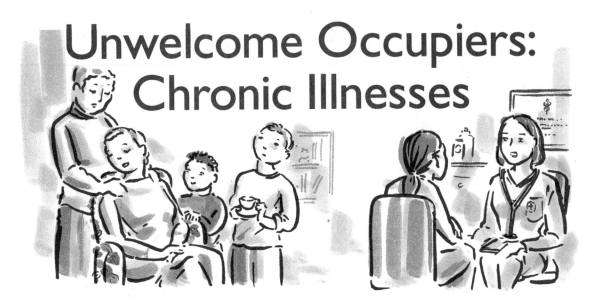

Chronic *adj.*: persistent, endless, lifelong. When a doctor says you have a chronic illness, that means it's here to stay.

Because a chronic illness has no cure, treating it requires a defensive strategy of tackling new symptoms when they appear and an offensive attack to slow the disease's progression.

"When a woman realizes that her illness is something that she has to live with for a long time—maybe even the rest of her life—she often feels helpless and powerless," says Debra S. Borys, Ph.D., assistant clinical professor of psychology at the University of California, Los Angeles. She may experience reactions ranging from denial, anger, and depression to grief over the loss of her health.

She will probably need to make permanent lifestyle changes to manage her illness. She may have to switch from a full-time job to a part-time one, learn to be content with a less-than-spotless house, and turn down invitations to go out with friends. All of these things can leave a woman feeling that she has lost control over her life.

Learning to Cope with a Chronic Illness

The good news is that you *can* feel in control of your life once again. To keep a positive attitude, view your illness as a new challenge and focus on the things that you can do, rather than the things you can't. "Deal with your illness like a project that has a bunch of tasks to be done," Dr. Borys suggests. Start by talking to your doctor and learning as much as you can about your illness. Here are some other "tasks" you can begin doing to cope with your condition.

Become a groupie. "Look for a support group that empowers you so you feel as though you've just been to an emotional filling station and now you're tanked up and ready to go out and accomplish things," says Orvalene Prewitt, cofounder and president of the National Chronic Fatigue Syndrome and Fibromyalgia Association.

Talking to others with the same illness provides tremendous emotional support. "Because everybody in the group shares a similar experience, there's a unique level of empathy," Dr. Borys says. You realize that you're not the only one going through this and you see that others have successfully progressed through the various stages of the disease.

Learn to surf. "If someone is confined to her home because of her illness, the Internet opens up the world to her," Dr. Borys says. You can find support groups on the 'net. And whether you're first learning about your illness or keeping up with the latest research, medical school Web sites are great places to turn for information.

Know your limits. As hard as it may be to accept, you probably need to take on less stress and physical activity than you used to, says Dr. Borys. Otherwise, you could end up worsening your condition. "Chances are, you can't accomplish as much—even on a good day—as you could when you didn't have your illness," she says.

Try a dose of laughter. There may be some truth to the familiar saying "Laughter is the best medicine." It turns out that laughing boosts your immune system, reduces stress, relaxes tense muscles, and improves oxygen and bloodflow to all parts of your body.

"When a comedian came to our support group, everyone so enjoyed his act that they sat there for 2 hours without getting up," Prewitt says. "That's really a feat for those with fibromyalgia, because sitting for long periods makes their muscles stiffen."

To add laughter to your life, read the comics

WOMEN ASK WHY

Why don't doctors make house calls anymore?

Visiting nurses—not doctors—make the majority of house calls these days. One reason for this change is the health-care system. Under managed care, doctors are pressured to see as many patients a day as they can, which leaves little time for house calls. What's more, the 12,900 family doctors who do still make house calls are not paid for their travel time.

House calls may no longer be standard practice, but they're especially important when a patient has a chronic or terminal illness. Doctors get to see how a person is being cared for. They can make sure that she's taking her medication and can learn what her environment is like—whether her room is cheery and well-ventilated or dark and stuffy. House calls also prevent patients who need a lot of care from spending all their time in doctors' offices. Not to mention that if a patient is frail or disabled, it may be easier and even safer for the doctor to come to her.

These things said, there are many times when house calls are not practical. If you think that you're having a heart attack, for example, many lifesaving procedures that are done at hospitals can't be done in your home.

Expert consulted
Barbara A. Majeroni, M.D.
Assistant professor of family medicine
State University of New York at Buffalo

section of the newspaper every day, rent a comedy movie once a week, and regularly see any friends whose humor you enjoy, Dr. Borys suggests.

Use mind over matter. Many people believe that the mind and body are connected and that a woman's thoughts can have an impact on her health. This belief is the basis for using visualization in healing—a tool that draws on one's inner strength to make one get well, says Judith Green, Ph.D., professor of psychology in the behavioral science department at Aims Community College in Greeley, Colorado, and a biofeedback therapist.

"Set aside 10 to 15 minutes a day for visualization," Dr. Green suggests. Start by relaxing both your mind and body. Sit in a quiet place, close your eyes, take a few deep breaths, and concentrate on emptying your mind of all your worries and to-do lists.

Then, use your mind to direct your body toward health. If you have asthma, for example, picture air filling your lungs with ease as you take each breath. If you have an autoimmune disease, such as lupus or multiple sclerosis, visualize your immune system working smoothly and your body being strong.

Take up tai chi. This gentle, slow-moving martial art may help women with chronic illnesses improve their physical conditions and sense of well-being. In one study, 19 patients with multiple sclerosis increased their walking speeds and flexibility after an 8-week class. They also developed more positive attitudes toward their conditions and were better able to handle their symptoms.

To find a tai chi instructor near you, check the yellow pages under "karate" or "martial arts" or call a martial arts school. While tai chi is generally regarded as safe for most conditions, you should check with your doctor before starting any exercise program. If you do experience increased pain while practicing tai chi, discontinue it.

WOMAN TO WOMAN

She Battles Her Chronic Illness with Blended Medicine and Optimism

Four years ago, mysterious symptoms left 22-year-old Jen Munn of Islip Terrace, New York, homebound and unable to work or socialize. Through a combination of conventional and alternative therapies, a positive attitude, and perseverance, she's now back on the path to improved health. Here's her story.

A few years ago, I was an active university student on my way to becoming a physician's assistant. On top of my course load, I lifted weights, took karate classes, rode an exercise bike, and swam twice a week. But when I was a sophomore, I always had the flu. I started getting leg pains and terrible back spasms. Even after cutting back on my workouts, the pains continued, and I was so exhausted that I'd go straight to bed after my classes. Then one morning, I woke up with the worst "flu" I'd ever had. I couldn't move, and my throat hurt so badly that I felt as if I had swallowed glass.

The doctors tested me for lupus, multiple sclerosis, Lyme disease, and epilepsy, but the tests came back negative. They put me on a bunch of antibiotics, but that didn't do the trick either.

Then, I started having tremendous difficulty reading. My eyes wouldn't follow the words, and I couldn't remember what I had read a few lines before. I had trouble speaking in complete sentences, had fainting spells, and was so weak that walking down a hallway was like running a marathon.

That's when I was diagnosed with chronic fatigue syndrome (CFS)—an illness with an unknown cause that has left

Making Everyday Tasks Easier

Wife. Mom. Career woman. Community volunteer. A woman does so many jobs in a day. But having a chronic illness can really cramp that superwoman style, making even routine

me disabled since 1996, just after graduation. I had to quit my new job and move home with my parents. For several months, I was so weak that my mom brought meals to my room; I couldn't even make it up the short flight of stairs to the kitchen.

As bad as things were, I didn't lose hope. I went from doctor to doctor until I found a CFS specialist. Now, I'm on medication to prevent the fainting spells, which are caused by a drastic drop in blood pressure when I stand for any period of time. I take a multivitamin and the mineral magnesium and give myself weekly B$_{12}$ injections for the fatigue. I'm always trying new supplements to find something that will help ease the symptoms even more. The herb feverfew helps relieve my severe headaches. I also use natural soap and shampoo to prevent the headaches and breathing problems I get from certain chemicals.

In the past few months, I've been well enough to take some short walks, and I've started lifting 2-pound hand weights when I feel up to it. That's a real feat, considering that I couldn't lift my hairbrush to my head a year ago.

I'm also able to spend less time in bed and more time on the computer. I'm trying to let other people know about CFS through a journal I keep on the Internet. I feel that it's worth sharing my personal experiences if it helps others realize that CFS is a very real and very serious disease.

For me, CFS is like a giant roadblock that I have to get through. Every month that I feel stronger, I'm a bit closer to tearing that roadblock down. Though I may never completely recover from CFS, my dream is to get well enough to live as normal a life as I can.

chores seem overwhelming. There are ways to maximize your energy and get things done with a small amount of effort.

Delegate household duties. Whether you're making dinner or washing a load of laundry, don't do it all on your own. Ask your kids and spouse to help. Have hubby carry that heavy basket of laundry.

If you live alone, reach out to your family, friends, or church. "For some people, it's hard to ask for help. But the truth is, a lot of people would be thrilled to give you a hand," Prewitt says.

Bring chores down to size. Large tasks such as cleaning the entire house can be quite daunting to someone with a chronic illness. If you break big tasks into several smaller ones, the job suddenly becomes much easier to handle, Dr. Borys says. Do a single, different task each day.

Stash a cleaning cart. "One woman in our support group put all of her cleaning supplies, a roll of paper towels, and a duster on a little roll-cart," Prewitt says. "That way, she didn't have to carry anything. She could quickly clean, and then hide the cart back in the closet—and still have some energy to spare."

Sit down on the job. Standing can be very draining for women who have chronic pain or fatigue. When cooking, try sitting on a stool to chop vegetables or mix ingredients, Prewitt suggests.

Give your diet a makeover. It's difficult for women with chronic illnesses to eat well because they have limited energy to prepare healthy meals. So they end up grabbing prepackaged foods. The problem is that these foods are often high in salt and fat and low in vitamins and minerals, says Kristine M. Napier, R.D., a registered dietitian in Cleveland and author of *Power Nutrition for Your Chronic Illness*. "Because of their poor diets, people with chronic

UNDERACTIVE THYROID

Chances are, you don't care much about your thyroid or what it does—unless it has stopped working.

This butterfly-shaped gland, located just below your Adam's apple, is involved in every organ system in your body. It produces two hormones that affect everything from the condition of your hair and skin to how fast your heart beats and your body metabolizes food, says Jacqueline Cohn, M.D., an endocrinologist practicing in Corpus Christi, Texas.

The most common form of thyroid disease is an underactive thyroid (also called hypothyroidism), which occurs when your thyroid stops producing enough hormones. As a result, you may start to feel sluggish, achy, fatigued, and depressed. You may also experience weight gain, constipation, sensitivity to cold, dry skin, hair loss, muscle cramps, joint stiffness, and increased menstrual flow.

Like many other chronic illnesses, hypothyroidism strikes women more often than men. As many as 1 in 10 women over age 65 have early signs of hypothyroidism—so Dr. Cohn recommends that women over 50 have their thyroids checked every 3 to 5 years. Any woman who has had more than one miscarriage should also have her thyroid checked because an underactive thyroid may be to blame for the miscarriages.

If left untreated, hypothyroidism can lead to high cholesterol and can increase your risk for heart disease.

Treating an underactive thyroid is straightforward. You simply take synthetic thyroid hormones, usually for the rest of your life. Once your doctor determines the correct dosage, you need to have your thyroid hormone levels rechecked only once a year.

illnesses are often marginally nourished." So they don't feel as well as they could. "Eating this way also puts them at risk for other illnesses, such as heart disease, osteoporosis, and cancer," she adds.

To break out of your bad eating habits, take advantage of the times when you have the most energy. If you typically feel your best in the afternoons, for example, prepare dinner then. Cook enough for more than one meal and freeze what you don't eat for another day.

Rework your work schedule. For some women, a career is a key part of their identities. It gives them satisfaction, fulfillment, and confidence. "One of women's biggest fears when they're diagnosed with a chronic illness is that they won't be able to work," Prewitt says. And some women do become so weak or disabled that they can't work.

"If working is important to your self-esteem and won't worsen your condition, figure out what you can do to make your job more suitable for you," Dr. Borys says. Perhaps you can cut back to part-time or work from home. If you have arthritis or fibromyalgia, for example, a more comfortable chair can make all the difference.

Defend Against the Defenders: Immune System Health

Sometimes, for no good reason, the world just seems to go haywire. Police arrest innocent people, a watchdog bites its owner, a miracle medicine ends up doing more harm than good. The very things we most trust betray us. If an event like this happens in the world we live in, we call it irony. If it happens inside the human body, we call it autoimmune disease.

Autoimmune diseases are complex illnesses, and their causes are unknown, but basically they all come down to one basic fact: Your own body treats you as if you were a stranger. Something goes haywire in your immune system, and the guardian cells designed to kill invaders, such as viruses, bacteria, and fungi, turn on and attack your own organs instead.

More than 80 illnesses fall into this category, and many seem to have an affinity for women, lupus perhaps most of all. More people have lupus than have AIDS, cerebral palsy, multiple sclerosis, sickle-cell anemia, and cystic fibrosis *combined*. That's enough people to fill the Sky-Dome in Toronto 25 times—and more than 90 percent of them are women.

Lupus can cause inflammation in several parts of your body, including your skin, joints, kidneys, heart, lungs, blood vessels, brain, and nervous system. But as frightening as that may sound, the bright reality is that 80 to 90 percent of people with lupus can live normal life spans if they follow the instructions of their physicians and take their medication as prescribed, says Michelle Petri, M.P.H., M.D., associate professor of medicine and director of the Lupus Center at Johns Hopkins University School of Medicine in Baltimore. That means close to two million people are finding ways to cope with and control their disease every day.

Risk Factors

What puts you at risk for lupus? Genetics, for one thing, Dr. Petri says. According to the Lupus Foundation of America, 10 percent of lupus patients have a parent or sibling who either has or may develop lupus, and 5 percent of children born to a parent with lupus will develop the disease.

Women who may be genetically predisposed to lupus often begin having symptoms as a result of some trigger. "Several clues lead us to believe that one important trigger is the female hormone estrogen," Dr. Petri says. Among the clues are the facts that 9 out of 10 lupus patients are women; it doesn't usually develop in women until after puberty, when estrogen is present; and birth control pills containing estrogen may precipitate the disease or worsen its symptoms in a few women.

Exposure to ultraviolet light is another common trigger. "Many women who are probably predisposed to lupus genetically don't actually have onset of the disease until they have a bad sunburn," Dr. Petri says. "A typical story I hear is that a woman comes back from a trip to Hawaii or the Caribbean with a high fever, a rash, and arthritis—and it turns out to be lupus."

Certain drugs and herbs may trigger lupus as well. Bactrim, a prescription medication, is one of them. "Some women have developed lupus after they were given this very common antibiotic, which is used all the time for urinary tract infections," Dr. Petri says. But prescription drugs aren't the only culprits. Echinacea, an herbal remedy commonly taken to boost the immune system to prevent or shorten colds, may also trigger lupus.

Other possible triggers include extreme stress, the hepatitis B vaccine, and the Epstein-Barr virus, Dr. Petri says.

Signs and Symptoms

The first symptoms of lupus often include fever, fatigue, and swollen or painful joints. If sun exposure triggered the disease, the heralding sign may be a red butterfly-shaped rash across your cheeks and nose. "The butterfly rash can occur for the first time after sun exposure and typically lasts for days or weeks," Dr. Petri says. Other symptoms include anemia, hair loss, mouth sores, chest pain when you breathe deeply

(pleurisy), fingers and toes that turn white or blue in the cold (Raynaud's phenomenon), seizures, swelling in your legs or ankles, and red raised patches called discoid lesions, which typically appear on your head, neck, or scalp.

Generally, there are three patterns of symptoms that women with lupus experience. Many women have flares every few months or so and usually need to take medication to bring the flares under control, Dr. Petri says. Other women always have active lupus and always need medication. And then there are some women with lupus who may go a few months to several years without experiencing a flare and are able to go off medication completely. These longer periods without symptoms are sometimes called remissions. "I'm hesitant to use the term *remission* because the lupus usually comes back," she says. "What's more, we really don't know why some patients have frequent flares and others can go off medication for long periods."

What exactly is a lupus flare? When new symptoms appear or the symptoms you already have worsen, you're having one. A number of things can cause a flare, including stress, sun exposure, or an infection.

If you suspect that a flare is developing, call your doctor right away. She may need to change your medications or dosages or take other steps to bring it under control, Dr. Petri says.

Don't Panic!

If you wake up one morning with a red rash on your face, don't jump to conclusions. The rash and lesions common in lupus can resemble a number of other skin conditions, including sunburn, contact dermatitis, vitiligo, psoriasis, or a combination of rosacea and seborrhea, says Marti Rothe, M.D., associate professor of dermatology and director of the Clinical Services and Phototherapy Center at the University of

Connecticut Health Center in Farmington. Or you may have discoid lupus, a type of lupus that affects only the skin.

Other common symptoms of lupus—joint pain, fatigue, and fever—are also signs of Lyme disease. If joint pain is your major complaint, arthritis may be the culprit, Dr. Petri says. If you're experiencing extreme fatigue, the cause could be anything from stress or a sleep disorder to an underactive thyroid or chronic fatigue syndrome.

Who Do I See?

If you have a rash or raised red patches on your skin, your best bet is to see a dermatologist. If she determines that it's lupus, she may refer you to a rheumatologist, a doctor who specializes in arthritis and other diseases of the bones, joints, and muscles.

If you have joint pain or other symptoms of lupus, you can see your family doctor or internist, a rheumatologist, or a clinical immunologist specializing in lupus. (Clinical immunologists treat immune system disorders.) To find a doctor in your area who is familiar with lupus, contact the Lupus Foundation of America, 1300 Piccard Drive, Suite 200, Rockville, MD 20850-4303.

What Can I Expect?

"It took 10 years of being sick and visits to 35 different doctors before I was finally diagnosed," says 41-year-

FIBROMYALGIA

About 30 percent of women with lupus also have a condition known as fibromyalgia. "We don't know why fibromyalgia is grossly overrepresented in women with lupus, especially since it's not an autoimmune or inflammatory disease," says Michelle Petri, M.P.H., M.D., associate professor of medicine and director of the Lupus Center at Johns Hopkins University School of Medicine in Baltimore.

Like lupus, fibromyalgia syndrome, or FMS, for short, affects women more often than men and is difficult to diagnose. There is no blood test or x-ray that confirms you have FMS, although your doctor may conduct such tests to rule out other conditions. The most common symptoms of FMS are chronic, widespread muscle pain or aches, fatigue, depression, sleep disturbances, and morning stiffness. Women with FMS have at least 11 of 18 possible tender points, found particularly in the neck, spine, shoulders, and hips, Dr. Petri explains. These points are very painful and sore when touched with a small amount of pressure.

As with lupus, women who have FMS may experience flare-ups and periods of remission. Women with FMS have low levels of certain natural hormones and chemicals in their brains and high levels of other chemicals. The cause of these abnormal levels is unknown.

FMS is generally treated with muscle relaxants and antidepressant drugs to relax muscles, improve sleep, and relieve depression. Injecting a local anesthetic or corticosteroids into particularly sore spots—a treatment known as triggerpoint injections—can help relieve pain. Doctors often recommend stretching and low-impact aerobic exercise, such as walking or swimming in a heated pool. Exercise both reduces muscle pain and improves fitness.

Some women with FMS find relief with alternative therapies such as acupuncture, physical therapy, chiropractic, and massage therapy. Alternative physicians may recommend vitamins, minerals such as magnesium, herbs such as St. John's wort, or other supplements such as malic acid, which is a substance found in apples. Check with your doctor before beginning any of these therapies or taking any supplements.

old Donna Manning of Agawam, Massachusetts. "I had a lot of joint pain, but my joints weren't always swollen. This caused doctors to think that the pain was in my head. Many doctors hinted that maybe I should seek psychiatric help. But I knew the pain was real."

This scenario is all too common. Some women experience symptoms for more than a year before they're diagnosed. Lupus often eludes doctors for two reasons. First, symptoms typically come on very gradually and may seem unrelated. If you have some joint stiffness, mild hair loss, fatigue, and mouth sores, that may not be enough to clue your doctor in to lupus, Dr. Petri says.

Second, there is no definitive diagnostic test. "The lupus blood test cannot by itself determine whether you have the disease because 10 to 20 percent of women who don't have lupus still test positive," Dr. Petri explains. If your lupus test, also called the antinuclear antibody test (ANA), is negative, it strongly suggests that you are disease-free. But if the ANA is positive, it's not sufficient to stop there and say that you have lupus, she says.

The ANA tests for certain antibodies with which your body attacks itself. If you test positive, your doctor should look for more clues by doing tests that check for other antibodies that work against your body and for blood levels of a group of proteins called *complement* that are often low in people who have active lupus. Your doctor may take other routine tests—including a skin biopsy, complete blood count, and urinalysis—and may check for kidney function or inflammation in your body.

But there is more to lupus than symptoms,

MULTIPLE SCLEROSIS

We've all heard about multiple sclerosis (MS). Perhaps you know someone with MS—a close friend, a neighbor, or a coworker. About 350,000 people in the United States have MS, most of them white women ages 20 to 50.

People with MS have multiple scarring (or sclerosis) in their brains and spinal cords, says Barbara S. Giesser, associate professor of clinical neurology at the Arizona Health Sciences Center in Tucson. These scars are areas where their nerves have been damaged. Healthy nerve fibers are like a roll of paper towels, she says. The nerve is the cardboard core protected by the layers of paper called the myelin sheath. In women with MS, the sheath is slowly stripped away by the body's own immune system. Left behind is scar tissue and, in some cases, an exposed nerve. As a result, nerve impulses traveling through the body are interrupted, much the way a phone connection can be muddled by static from a thunderstorm. These muddled messages cause people with MS to experience pain, difficulty walking, numbness or tingling in their arms and legs, loss of balance, muscle weakness, bladder-control problems, eye pain or blurred vision, slurred speech, and problems thinking or remembering.

Dr. Giesser adds that it is becoming clear through research that not only the myelin sheath but the nerve fiber itself is damaged in MS. This nerve fiber damage is thought to be an important cause of long-term disability and problems with thinking processes that can occur with MS.

tests, and treatments. Women ride a roller coaster of emotions after they find out they're sick. At first, they may have a sense of validation because their illness has a name and is not all in their heads. They may be afraid that they won't be able to work or that they may even die. Some women don't know what to tell their families, friends, and coworkers. And it's common for them to feel depressed over the loss of their normal lifestyles.

"I was 24 years old when I was diagnosed

Diagnosing MS is difficult because there is no one test that proves a person has it, and some symptoms could be caused by other diseases.

MS is considered an autoimmune disease, but the cause of the self-attack is unknown. There does seem to be a genetic link, since a person's risk of developing MS significantly increases if she has a close family member with the disease. But genetics don't appear to be the only factor. Researchers have also been studying various bacteria and viruses, thinking that perhaps an infectious agent triggers MS.

Most people with MS go through cycles of relapse and remission and are able to lead productive lives, although they may have some degree of disability, Dr. Giesser says. Overall, women have a 50-50 chance of walking without assistance 15 years after diagnosis, and 85 percent of MS patients have normal life expectancies, she says.

Treatment is aimed at slowing the destruction of the myelin sheath and managing symptoms. Drugs such as corticosteroids are used to reduce the inflammation that occurs when the immune system attacks the nerve fibers, Dr. Giesser says. Other drugs, called immunomodulators, are used to slow down that attack. And still other drugs are prescribed to help decrease pain, fatigue, depression, and bladder and bowel dysfunction. Physical therapy, occupational therapy, and speech therapy can help women improve their ability to do day-to-day tasks, Dr. Giesser says.

with lupus. At that time, the prognosis for patients was not as hopeful as it is today," recalls Lynda Puglisi of Denver, who was diagnosed with lupus 13 years ago. "I remember going to a support group meeting, and the people there asked my family, 'Who's going to take her in, because she's not going to be able to take care of herself?' It terrified me to not know what was happening to my body, and I remember having the image in my mind that I was not going to have a normal life."

Many women go through a period where they feel helpless or hopeless and may ask, "Why me?" Dr. Petri says. "It's important that your doctor address these emotions and tell you the good news: We're doing so well with our current therapies that patients should have great hope that they will be able to have a normal life."

Conventional Wisdom

If you have lupus, chances are that you'll be taking some kind of medication regularly, even if it's just ibuprofen for joint pain and inflammation. Here are some of the most common medications as well as the steps you can take to prevent flares.

Shun the sun. Before you had lupus, it may have felt great to bask in the sun and darken your tan. But now, those ultraviolet rays can wreak havoc on your skin, and some women are so sensitive to sunlight that just 10 minutes of exposure could send them into a flare. For that reason, doctors recommend that women with lupus stay out of the sun as much as possible, especially between the peak hours of 10:00 A.M. and 2:00 P.M. When you do venture outdoors in the daytime, be sure to wear sunscreen with an SPF of 30 and with UVA protection, Dr. Rothe advises. And don't skip the sunscreen if it's cold or cloudy outside. The rays that bring on lupus flares are still present when there's heavy cloud cover or if it's wintertime. So put on your sunscreen every time you go outside during the day.

Also keep in mind that sunscreen wears off after a while. "Make sure that you reapply sunscreen every 4 hours," Dr. Rothe says. "Reapply sooner if you're sweating or swimming." In addition to wearing sunscreen, it's a good idea to cover up if you go outside.

Dr. Rothe warns that you also need to be wary of windows. Neither windows nor windshields block the harmful rays that aggravate lupus.

Take your temp. One common symptom of lupus is a fever. In fact, some women with lupus have a low-grade fever most of the time. But a fever that's higher than normal could be a sign of infection or of a lupus flare.

Women with lupus are more prone to infections, and certain drugs used to treat the illness can increase the risk even more because they suppress the immune system. "That's why I advise my patients to take their temperature when they're not feeling well," Dr. Petri says. "If they have a temperature above 101°F, I tell them to contact me or another physician immediately. Because if they have an infection, we need to find and treat it quickly."

Take a shot. Because women with lupus are more susceptible to infections, they need to get certain vaccinations routinely. "It's very important for them to be protected against common infections, including influenza and pneumococcus," Dr. Petri says. Lupus patients should get the flu shot every October and the pneumonia shot every 5 years, she recommends.

One shot they should not get is the hepatitis B vaccine. "Recently, there has been some concern that the hepatitis B vaccine may have triggered lupus in some susceptible patients, although it has never been proven conclusively," Dr. Petri says. "Right now, we're recommending that lupus patients hold off until we have better studies."

WOMEN ASK WHY

Why does my doctor always interrupt me when I'm explaining what's wrong with me?

Here's the diagnosis: Your doctor appears to be suffering from poor-listening-skills-itis. The most effective treatment in cases like this is for you to consider finding another doctor. Your health is a very precious thing. You wouldn't take your best evening gown to a dry cleaner whom you didn't trust. You need to treat yourself with the same respect and find a doctor with whom you feel comfortable. At the very least, a doctor who interrupts you makes you feel as if she doesn't care about you as a person. At worst, your doctor may be missing valuable information because she's cutting you off before you're finished telling her what's wrong.

If you decide to look for a new doctor, make sure the physician you choose takes the time to listen to you and welcomes any questions you have. I encourage my patients to write down their questions and concerns and bring them to the appointment.

Take your meds. Your doctor will probably use a combination of prescription and nonprescription medications to treat your various symptoms, Dr. Petri says. One class of drugs used for lupus are nonsteroidal anti-inflammatory drugs (NSAIDs), such as ibuprofen and naproxen (Aleve). These drugs help reduce inflammation, and some are available over the counter.

Corticosteroids such as prednisone are a more potent class of drugs prescribed to reduce inflammation. You can take these by mouth, by injection, or in creams that you rub onto your skin.

Drugs called antimalarials, which were developed to treat malaria, are helpful for relieving lupus symptoms such as fatigue, joint pain, and

And you shouldn't be the only one asking questions—your doctor should have questions as well. To truly treat your problem, it's important for the doctor to go beyond the symptoms and get to know you, the person. If you're having frequent headaches, for example, your doctor should ask questions such as "What kind of work do you do?" and "What is your family life like?" Your headaches may be caused by stress, depression, allergies, or even a change in your vision. Many doctors will treat the headache, not the person. As a result, the headaches may continue because the root of the problem has not been addressed.

To find the right doctor for you, ask your friends, neighbors, or coworkers whether their doctors take the time to listen and to probe for the causes of their problems. Your health is worth the effort to find a doctor who's more attentive to your needs.

Expert consulted
Gloria Walker, M.D.
Family practitioner
Tree Heart Holistic Center
Cincinnati

skin rashes. Antimalarials such as chloroquine (Aralen) or hydroxychloroquine (Plaquenil) may even prevent future flares.

For more serious cases of lupus, a doctor may prescribe drugs such as methotrexate (Mexate), azathioprine (Imuran), or cyclophosphamide (Cytoxan). These drugs slow the progression of lupus by suppressing the immune system and by weakening its attack on your body's own systems.

As with most drugs, these medications can cause a number of side effects. Your doctor should discuss all the possibilities with you, Dr. Petri says.

Look to the future. Research to find new therapies for lupus is under way at several universities and medical centers as well as at the National Institutes of Health. Among the most promising treatments being tested is a vaccine that inhibits T cells. This treatment actually teaches the immune system not to attack itself. "The advantage is that you prevent the targeting of self, but you don't impair your body's ability to fight infection," says Bevra Hahn, M.D., who is conducting T cell research at the University of California, Los Angeles, School of Medicine, where she is professor of medicine and chief of rheumatology.

These treatments have been successful in rodents with lupus, and some are now being tested on people. They may be virtually free of side effects and would be helpful not only for lupus but also for other autoimmune diseases such as multiple sclerosis and rheumatoid arthritis, Dr. Hahn says.

Research is also being done to find out whether the male hormone DHEA is a safe and effective treatment for mild lupus.

Great Alternatives

When your body is coping with a chronic illness like lupus, it needs all the help it can get. From eating a balanced diet to getting enough rest, living a healthy lifestyle is paramount to keeping your body in the best possible shape. These lifestyle tips from alternative practitioners may help prevent lupus flares and offer relief from common lupus symptoms.

Skimp on fat. The major cause of death in lupus patients is not lupus at all. "It's heart disease," says Dr. Petri, "which they tend to develop 30 years earlier than other women." This is due

WOMEN ASK WHY

Why do I feel even more tired after spending several days in bed resting?

That depends on why you were in bed in the first place. If you were resting to get over a respiratory infection, for example, you may still feel tired because fatigue is one of the symptoms of such an illness. Even though you may feel better, it could take a few weeks for the fatigue to subside. If you've been in bed with a stomach virus, you may feel tired, weak, and dizzy from dehydration. When you're unable to eat or drink because of nausea, you can lose fluids and electrolytes, and that makes you feel sluggish. To wipe out the fatigue, make sure that you drink at least eight 8-ounce glasses of fluids a day.

You may also feel weak and tired from muscle deconditioning. That's when your muscles become out of shape because they haven't been used for a while. Deconditioning starts to happen after just a few days of lying around. The longer you're in bed, the more deconditioning you'll have. Once you get back into your normal routine for a couple of weeks, your muscles will become conditioned once again, and the fatigue should go away.

If you have been doing your regular routine for several weeks and you still have fatigue, go see your doctor. You may have a treatable condition that's causing your fatigue such as a viral infection, an underactive thyroid, anemia, or depression.

Expert consulted
Ellen S. Mitchell, R.N., Ph.D.
Associate professor
University of Washington School of Nursing
Seattle

to an acceleration of hardening of the arteries, she explains.

A low-fat diet can help prevent heart disease. It may also help prevent lupus flares, says Kristine M. Napier, R.D., a registered dietitian in Cleveland who has had lupus for 18 years. "I recommend that women with lupus get only 15 to 20 percent of their calories from fat," says Napier, who is also the author of *Power Nutrition for Your Chronic Illness*.

Load up on fruits and vegetables. When you go to the grocery store, park your shopping cart in the produce section and fill it up. Fruits and vegetables are chock-full of antioxidants, which have been found to reduce a person's risk of developing the autoimmune disease rheumatoid arthritis and may be helpful for lupus as well, Napier says. Shoot for 10 servings of fruits and vegetables a day.

Sprinkle on flaxseed. A food from nature called flaxseed has been found to reverse some forms of kidney disease—one of the more serious complications of lupus, Napier says. Flaxseed may help lupus because it contains phytoestrogens and omega-3 fatty acids, which help reduce the inflammation of blood vessels that can lead to kidney problems. Add the flax to your diet gradually until you're eating 2 to 4 tablespoons a day. Sprinkle flaxseed on hot or cold cereal or add it to salad or yogurt. Flaxseed is available at most health food stores. Just make sure that you get the ground or milled form, Napier says, because the whole seeds pass through the body undigested. If you heat or cook the flaxseed, it will not lose its potency, she adds. Store it in an airtight container in the fridge for maximum freshness. Take it with at least 8 ounces of water.

Reel in relief. Fish such as tuna, salmon, herring, and mackerel are high in the same helpful omega-3's found in flaxseed, Napier says. To help reduce the inflammation caused by lupus, try to include two to four servings of fish in your diet every week.

Bone up on calcium. Prednisone (Deltasone)—one of the most common drugs used in treating lupus—causes women to lose bone mass because it interferes with calcium absorption, Dr. Petri says. As a result, women who are taking prednisone are prone to developing osteoporosis, a condition in which your bones become so weak and brittle that they easily break.

Women with lupus who are on corticosteroids such as prednisone should get 2,000 milligrams of calcium and 800 IU of vitamin D every day through diet and supplements, says Napier.

Care for your joints. A compound from the sea and another from a common fruit can help relieve arthritis pain in women with lupus. Glucosamine sulfate—found in the shells of crabs, lobsters, and shrimp—helps rebuild cartilage in joints damaged by arthritis, says Stacey Raffety, R.N., N.D., a licensed acupuncturist and naturopathic physician practicing in Tigard, Oregon. Take 500 milligrams three times a day, she recommends.

To help relieve joint inflammation and pain, Dr. Raffety suggests that you also take an enzyme called bromelain, which is found in pineapple. "I recommend trying to get 900 to 1,800 milligrams of bromelain every day. Divide the total daily amount into four mini-doses and take one dose a half-hour before eating breakfast and dinner and another dose 1 to 2 hours after eating these meals," she advises. Bromelain may cause nausea, vomiting, diarrhea, skin rashes, and heavy menstrual bleeding, and it may increase the risk of bleeding in people taking aspirin or blood thinners. Don't take it if you are allergic to pineapple.

Reduce your fatigue. Some women with lupus may find themselves experiencing insomnia at night and then feeling very fatigued during the day. "It's quite possible that their adrenal glands have been depleted of the natural hormone cortisol that helps direct sleep patterns," Dr. Raffety says. A stressful event, such as a chronic illness, is what typically depletes a person's adrenal glands.

"To support and heal the adrenal glands, I recommend that patients take a 50-milligram B complex with extra B_5 (pantothenic acid) once a day and drink three cups of licorice tea a day," Dr. Raffety adds. If you have kidney disease, check with your doctor before drinking licorice tea.

To make the tea, use 1 tablespoon of fresh herb per cup, steep it for 10 minutes, strain, and drink. It takes awhile for adrenal glands to heal—some women start to feel better in a couple of months, and others take years, says Dr. Raffety. Don't use licorice if you have diabetes, high blood pressure, liver or kidney disorders, or low potassium levels. Don't use it daily for more than 4 to 6 weeks, because overuse can lead to water retention, high blood pressure caused by potassium loss, or impaired heart and kidney function.

Bank your energy. Another way to manage your fatigue is to plan your days and weeks wisely so that you can reserve your energy for when you need it most. If you know you're going out one evening, for example, take a nap that afternoon so you'll still have enough energy to go out, Dr. Petri suggests. If you tend to have more energy in the morning, do your household chores then or schedule any appointments for the A.M. hours.

Work out. Exercising may be the last thing you feel like doing when you have the pain and fatigue that come with lupus, but it's crucial for women with lupus to exercise regularly, for several reasons, Dr. Petri says. First, exercise helps prevent the muscle weakness that results from prolonged periods of inactivity. Second, it can help prevent osteoporosis and weight gain, two common side effects of taking prednisone and of being inactive. Regular exercise will improve your cardiovascular fitness, which will lower your risk for heart disease. Physical activity also reduces stress and joint stiffness.

If you haven't been exercising, check with your doctor before starting an exercise program. If you get your doc's okay, start slowly, gradually increasing the duration and intensity of your exercise. "I started with the step machine. I would do it for only 15 minutes, but it felt like days because the fatigue was so strong," Puglisi says. "For me, exercise was really the key to my recovery. Once I started doing that, I began to feel better and better."

Try to work up to exercising for 30 minutes 5 or 6 days a week, Dr. Hahn says. Many women with lupus are able to swim and walk because these activities don't put a lot of stress on their joints, Dr. Petri says.

Wash away pain. Warm-water therapy, such as a whirlpool bath, can help soothe the joint and muscle pain common with lupus. "When I'm having a flare, I'll sit in our whirlpool bath. The swirling water is very therapeutic for pain," says Kate Purcell, R.N., a nurse recruiter in Oklahoma City who has had lupus for 8 years.

If you don't have a whirlpool bathtub or jacuzzi in your home, take a hot shower or place a heating pad covered in a thin towel on a particularly sore spot for 20 minutes, Dr. Petri suggests.

Try hands-on therapy. Some women with lupus find that acupuncture or massage can help relieve stress and decrease joint and muscle pain. Look for a licensed acupuncturist or a certified massage therapist—or recruit your spouse, child, or friend. "When I'm really hurting, I'll ask my husband, Jim, to give me a massage. He has that magic hand. He knows not to rub so hard that it hurts me more," Purcell says.

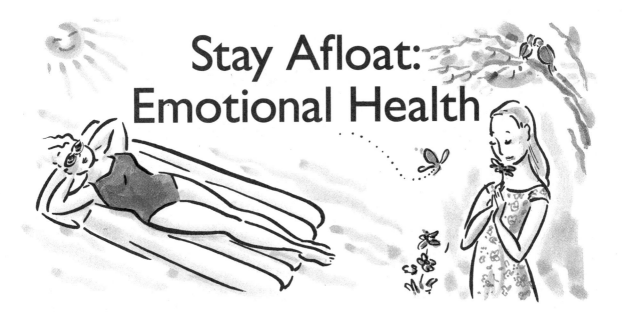

Stay Afloat: Emotional Health

Marilyn Monroe struggled with it. So did Tammy Wynette. Natalie Wood and Princess Diana both fought to resist it. Even Carmen Miranda, singing Brazilian sambas with a smile on her face and a basket of fruit on her head, had to fight against its smothering pall.

Depression. It's so widespread that it's sometimes called the common cold of mental illness. One out of every four women will have a bout of major depression during her lifetime. That means she'll have feelings of sadness and despair, inconsolable misery, and guilt that last for more than 2 weeks and interfere with her work, her relationships, and even her eating and sleeping.

Some women will face a different challenge: a milder but longer-lasting form of depression called dysthymia (a Greek word meaning "ill humor"), which can make life seem dull, gray, and continually sad. It generally goes on for more than 2 years and may end up developing into full-blown depression.

Unlike the common cold, however, depression can't have its way with you if you don't want it to. You have an effective storehouse of weapons that you can use to fight back.

Risk Factors

A woman whose mother or father suffered from depression is two to three times more likely than normal to become depressed herself, so a family history of depression is obviously a strong risk factor. But women accumulate even stronger risk factors during their lives that have nothing to do with genetics.

For example, three out of four people who develop depression can trace it to some major stress point in their lives—the death of a spouse, the loss of a job, a divorce, or an illness. "It's not uncommon for people who are seriously ill to be depressed, and sometimes their depression goes undiagnosed," says Carol Landau, Ph.D., professor of psychiatry and behavior at Brown University School of Medicine in Providence, Rhode Island. "And although they have good reasons to feel sad and depressed, clinical depression is a serious illness." They need treatment. "Treatment improves your quality of life, no matter what. It can help you see that, even when things are rough, you do have some choices in your life," she adds.

Another high-risk group comprises women who say that they are in unhappy, unsupportive marriages. They are 25 times more likely to be depressed than women who say that they are happily married, suggesting that a stressful relationship may be a much stronger risk factor than family history. But that doesn't mean bad relationships necessarily cause depression, says Bonnie Strickland, Ph.D., professor of psychology at the University of Massachusetts at Amherst. "Women who are already depressed may be more likely to perceive the negative side of their relationships. Or they may be choosing inappropriate partners. Or depression may exacerbate the stress of marriage. It's certainly a question that needs to be addressed."

Finally, having had one episode of depression greatly increases your risk of having another. "Without appropriate treatment, about half of the women who are clinically depressed will experience another episode or more," says Dr. Strickland.

Prevention

As with any illness, avoiding depression altogether is far preferable to having to fight your way from its dark night of the soul. While there is no way to guarantee that you'll never become severely depressed, you may be able to lower your risk.

First of all, look after your general health. That means get enough sleep, eat nutritious meals, and exercise regularly. "Your brain is part of your body, so keeping your body healthy is keeping your brain healthy," says Peg Nopoulos, M.D., assistant professor in the department of psychiatry at the University of Iowa in Iowa City.

Medical illnesses often run hand in hand with depression, says Michelle Nostheide, a social worker at the National Mental Health Association in Alexandria, Virginia. So living a healthy lifestyle should be your number one priority.

Your number two priority should be to live an active lifestyle. Do you like riding roller coasters? Is spending hours at museums your idea of a good time? Doing the things you like to do and surrounding yourself with people who enjoy doing them with you will help you feel good about yourself, Nostheide says. So be active in the world. Be curious, get involved, read. The more productive you are, the better chance you'll have of preventing depression.

Once you start feeling symptoms of depression, however, such as changes in sleep patterns, changes in your appetite, difficulty concentrating, fatigue or loss of energy, or feelings of worthlessness and helplessness, see a professional, recommends Dr. Nopoulos. Don't expect to be able to cure yourself, she says, just as you wouldn't expect to treat yourself for bronchitis.

Signs and Symptoms

There are many levels to depression, from mild, which allows you to function in more or less normal fashion, to severe, which causes deep and persistent feelings of sadness or despair that interfere with your work, friendships, family life, and physical health.

Not only do severely depressed people tend to feel helpless and hopeless but they also tend to blame themselves for having these feelings. They may sleep fitfully, or they may sleep too much. They may lose their appetites, or they may overeat. But no matter how the symptoms manifest themselves, depressed women tend to feel overwhelmed and exhausted, and they may stop participating in certain everyday activities altogether, says Ellen Leibenluft, M.D., chairperson of the unit for affective disorders in the pediatrics and developmental neuropsychiatry branch at the National Institute of Mental Health in Bethesda, Maryland. Some may also have thoughts of death or suicide. (For more information, see "Suicide: An Epidemic among Women?" on page 134.)

Don't Panic!

Keep in mind that everyone feels sad on occasion. It's natural and emotionally healthy to grieve over upsetting events. These feelings of grief can be extreme, but they tend to become less intense on their own as time goes on. "Allowing yourself to recognize and express all your emotions, whether it's sadness, anger, hope, or happiness, lets you be authentic," Dr. Strickland says. "It can enhance your connection with others and increase self-esteem." Sadness is not self-absorbing or isolating in the way depression is.

Also, keep in mind that even if you are depressed, most depression can be successfully treated. "With the recent advances in both psychotherapy and antidepressant medication, there is always hope, no matter how hopeless it feels," Dr. Landau says.

Who Do I See?

If you have a family doctor, you can certainly see or call her to tell her your concerns. Some family doctors have experience treating depression, and those who don't will most likely refer you to a psychiatrist. Psychiatrists are able to prescribe medications for depression, and many also provide psychotherapy, or talk therapy.

BIPOLAR DISORDER

All of us have our ups and downs, but people with bipolar disorder have higher ups and lower downs. They have periods of depression, with its typical symptoms, and periods of mania. Mania often appears as an expansive or irritable mood, inflated self-esteem, little need for sleep, talkativeness, distractibility, or a tendency to do pleasurable things that can have painful consequences, such as going on expensive shopping sprees or having an extramarital affair. Some forms of bipolar disorder also cause agitation, paranoia, hallucinations, or rage. Most people with bipolar disorder have plenty of "normal" time in between periods of depression or mania.

Like depression, bipolar disorder is caused by an imbalance of brain chemistry, and it can run in families. It's usually treated with drugs. Lithium remains a popular "antimanic" drug, but other, newer drugs also can help; so may some antidepressants and antipsychotics. Keeping a regular schedule that includes regular times for sleep and exercise and avoiding caffeine, alcohol, marijuana, or other mood-altering drugs can also help.

You can also talk about your problems and learn new ways to approach them with a psychologist or a licensed clinical social worker. Many women with depression who need medication will go to see both a psychiatrist and a psychologist, who work closely together on her case.

What Can I Expect?

Everyone's experience of depression is different. You may not realize that you're depressed but may go to your regular family doctor because of bothersome symptoms such as general fatigue or vague aches and pains. Getting an accurate diagnosis may very well be the first step to feeling better. "For most people, it's a relief to get a name and label on what they are experiencing," Dr. Strickland says.

Your doctor may prescribe antidepressants, but don't expect immediate results. They take time to work, and sometimes you'll have to try several medications before you find the one that's right for you. "You can't really know if a drug is going to work for you until you've taken it for 8 or even 12 weeks," Dr. Leibenluft says. Women who are so depressed that they're suicidal may be hospitalized for part of this time. And those who are anxious as well as depressed might be given a faster-acting tranquilizer, such as alprazolam (Xanax).

How long you'll need to take these drugs depends in part on your medical history, Dr. Leibenluft says. "Usually, if you've had two or more previous episodes of depression, especially if they were severe, your doctor may recommend that you take antidepressants for a longer time." So some people go on and off antidepressants, while some stay on them for years. Sometimes, a drug that has worked well for a few years stops working or doesn't work as well as it did previously, and your psychiatrist may try switching drugs or combining them.

Conventional Wisdom

These days, more and more women who are depressed are given antidepressant medications. That's because these drugs have proved helpful for many people. "It may be necessary to correct chemical imbalances in the brain that cause depression," says Dr. Leibenluft.

There are many antidepressant drugs on the market, and your doctor will ask you lots of

SUICIDE: AN EPIDEMIC AMONG WOMEN?

As with many things, women who attempt suicide do it differently from their male counterparts. Men are more likely to choose violent, irreversible means—using a gun or jumping from a high window—while women prefer drug-and-alcohol combinations, drug overdoses, or carbon monoxide poisoning. Women are about twice as likely as men to attempt suicide but are less likely to complete the deed. They may stop or be discovered before they are dead.

Women with untreated severe depression are at high risk. And among those being treated for severe depression, the time of highest risk is during the first 3 weeks after hospitalization, says Rhoda Olkin, Ph.D., professor of clinical psychology at the California School of Professional Psychology in Alameda.

"People who are severely depressed often don't have the wherewithal to kill themselves," she explains. "It's when the depression starts to be slightly alleviated that people have the energy to try to make the attempt."

Most people are suicidal for no longer than 48 hours at a time, although several such periods may pass before a person pulls out of the mood altogether.

Signs that someone is contemplating suicide may include the following:

Tuning out or turning off. She becomes withdrawn and uncommunicative.

questions about your symptoms and general health to determine the antidepressant that seems right for you. About 60 to 70 percent of the people who can tolerate the side effects of antidepressants get better with the first drug they take. Some will need to try a second antidepressant and some, rarely, a third.

Psychotherapy has traditionally also been considered a part of treatment for depression. But in these days of managed care, a woman is lucky if her health insurance pays for more than a few sessions of therapy, says Dr. Strickland. So psychologists scramble to find something that can

Making final arrangements. She begins putting her affairs in order, giving things away, changing her will, or talking about going away.

Risk taking or self-destructive behavior. She may start doing things that could easily end in injury. Reckless driving is a good example.

Sudden elevated mood. A sudden change in mood from gloomy to sunny can precede a suicide attempt.

Direct or indirect statements about suicide. It's not true that people who talk about suicide never do it. They do. Even jokes about suicide should be taken seriously.

Ask her, "Are you thinking of suicide?" Contrary to popular belief, you aren't putting ideas into a person's head. You may have opened the door to honest communication and voiced your concerns.

Then ask, "Do you have a plan? A method? A means? When were you planning to do it?" Concrete plans indicate an immediate crisis.

If it seems to you that someone you know is contemplating suicide, do not leave the person alone, says Dr. Olkin. Take charge, offer support, make sure that she has no means available to hurt herself. If it appears to be an emergency, take her to a crisis center, a hospital emergency room, a mental health center, her psychiatrist, or her family doctor.

thought patterns, including automatic negative thoughts that can influence your mood. You'll learn how to change them."

In the course of interpersonal therapy, you'll discuss your personal and social interactions with others and see how they are having an impact on your mood. Basically, you'll work on improving relationships so that you'll feel better about yourself. Research has shown that both cognitive-behavioral and interpersonal psychotherapy are effective treatments for depression.

Great Alternatives

Women who do more than just take drugs to treat their depression often do better in the long run. They learn how to provide balance, perspective, and meaning in their lives. Here are some additional suggestions for keeping depression at bay.

Cultivate a confidante. One classic sociology study, done in the slums of London, found that among women, the outstanding protective factor against depression was having a close confidante, someone to whom they could express any emotion. "It's this freedom to express a full range of emotions—any kind of emotions—that therapists believe sustains mental health," says Rhoda Olkin, Ph.D., professor of clinical psychology at the California School of Professional Psychology in Alameda.

Create a distraction. Men do this more than women do, and it tends to inoculate them against depression, Dr. Olkin says. Of course, a man's way of distracting himself could be hanging out at the corner barroom, which simply substitutes another problem. Women, in-

help in a short period of time, such as cognitive-behavioral psychotherapy, interpersonal psychotherapy, or combinations of the two.

"You're not likely to lie around on a couch talking about your childhood," Dr. Strickland says. "You will try to change your behavior and improve your mood in the present rather than dwelling in the past. In cognitive-behavioral therapy, you'll talk about what you want to change now and how you might do that. The psychologist will want to know what makes you happy and the conditions that lead you to be depressed. You'll examine your behaviors and

MY MAMA TOLD ME

Why are women more likely than men to get depressed?

Women are twice as likely as men to be depressed, but no one knows why.

Some experts say that women's nervous and hormonal systems respond to life's stressors differently from men's. Some say, too, that women are socialized to repress anger, so they learn to get sad, not mad. That's one reason assertiveness training, which helps women deal effectively with anger-provoking situations, is sometimes part of psychotherapy.

In addition, women are socialized to put on happy faces and take responsibility for the emotional well-being of others, including husbands and children. When things don't go well within their families, women may blame themselves and brood about what they believe are their shortcomings.

Finally, men may simply display their dark moods differently. Some researchers believe that men who are having problems with alcoholism, violence, or other self-destructive behaviors are actually depressed and would benefit from treatment.

So if you count all the guys down at the corner bar or driving around in pickup trucks with cases of beer behind the seats, the numbers actually come out about even.

Expert consulted
Bonnie Strickland, Ph.D.
Professor of psychology
University of Massachusetts
Amherst

like, and do them even if you don't feel up to it, Dr. Olkin says. "That will start a positive motion that moves into other areas of your life."

Check your medicine chest. Some medications can cause depression. Among the most common are beta-blockers, used to reduce high blood pressure; a class of antibiotics called quinolones (Levaquin is one); steroid drugs, used for autoimmune diseases (these can cause both depression and mania); large doses of any kind of anti-inflammatory, as might be used to treat rheumatoid arthritis; and benzodiazepine tranquilizers, which are often prescribed to women and include alprazolam (Xanax) and diazepam (Valium). Ask your doctor about the chances that a drug you're taking might be causing your depression. He may be able to switch you to a similarly acting drug that does not have a depressing effect.

Ask your doctor about St. John's wort. This depression-relieving herb has become popular in the last few years. Its main active ingredient, hypericin, helps to regulate levels of the mood-lifting brain chemical serotonin, just like some antidepressant drugs, such as fluoxetine (Prozac), paroxetine (Paxil), and sertraline (Zoloft). But there are some things that you need to know to use St. John's wort safely and effectively. It is not recommended for treatment of severe depression, bipolar disorder (manic-depression), or disorders that involve hallucinations and suicidal thoughts.

Don't take it if you are already taking a prescription antidepressant or other psychoactive

stead, tend to brood over their problems. "Learning to distract yourself is actually a part of cognitive-behavioral therapy," Dr. Olkin explains.

Exercise is an ideal distraction, but a good book or movie, a favorite hobby, or a pet can work just as well. Do things you like or used to

drugs. Occasional side effects may include agitation, sleep loss, and increased sensitivity to the sun, which can result in sunburn.

Look for a standardized alcohol-derived extract (the alcohol has been removed) containing 0.3 percent hypericin. Experts usually suggest a typical dose of 300 milligrams three times a day. Expect to wait 4 to 6 weeks before noticing an improvement. It's best to take St. John's wort only with knowledgeable medical supervision.

Fill your exercise prescription. Studies show that regular exercise can work as well as psychotherapy at relieving mild to moderate depression, says Kate Hays, Ph.D., author of *Working It Out: Using Exercise in Psychotherapy.* Try walking, running, or weight lifting for a minimum of 20 minutes, three times a week, she says. Exercise may have both an immediate and a long-term biochemical influence on your mood.

If you simply can't motivate yourself to exercise, try doing a physical activity that you enjoy, and approach it slowly but steadily, says Dr. Strickland.

Load up on fatty fish. The omega-3 fatty acids found in fish oils may help ease the symptoms of bipolar disorder, according to a preliminary study from researchers at McLean Hospital in Belmont, Massachusetts. The fatty acids may inhibit transmission of brain signals that trigger dramatic mood swings that characterize the disorder. The participants in the study took about 10 grams a day of fish oil from capsules.

Fish-oil capsules can cause nosebleeds and easy bruising, however. Don't take them if you have a bleeding disorder, uncontrolled high blood pressure, or diabetes; if you take anticoagulants (blood thinners) or use aspirin regularly; or if you are allergic to any kind of fish. Do not substitute with fish-liver oil, because it is high in vitamins A and D, which are toxic in high amounts.

Connect with the larger whole. Depression can be a signal that you have disconnected from the natural world and the soul nourishment that it can provide, says Sarah A. Conn, Ph.D., a lecturer on psychology at Harvard Medical School and founder of the Ecopsychology Institute of the Center for Psychology and Social Change in Cambridge, Massachusetts. To reconnect, she says, start by spending 5 to 10 minutes a day with "a natural being." This can be a tree, a plant, a grassy corner in a park, even clouds or a view out a window. "Simply observe; pay attention to changes," she says. "Then, start to address your deeper questions: 'What does my heart desire? How can I honor that desire? How does it connect me with the world? How does it invite me into the world?'" The natural world becomes an object of meditation that allows your inner world to emerge, she says.

Tune in to natural rhythms. Depression can also be a symptom of being so caught up in the speed of today's consumer-oriented society that you forget how to slow down, Dr. Conn says. "If we develop an ongoing relationship with the natural world, we can learn a lot about natural rhythms and the way we fit into nature." This might include adjusting your sleep patterns to follow the setting and rising of the sun, walking short distances rather than driving, caring for a garden, or just sitting and being still.

Shed some light on the problem. People who get sluggish and irritable during the winter months may actually have seasonal affective disorder (SAD), a form of depression or bipolar disorder that can be relieved with medications and exposure to real or simulated sunlight, says Dr. Leibenluft. People with SAD usually feel their worst in January and February, when days are already lengthening again, and perk up by March or April. To counteract the effects, take a 45-minute stroll in the morning or at lunchtime. Sunlight-

CAN SAM-e SUPPLEMENTS MAKE YOU SMILE?

It almost sounds too good to be true. A hot, new nutritional supplement being used for depression, S-adenosylmethionine—or SAM-e (Sammy), for short—promises to work faster than antidepressants, have minimal side effects, and provide other health benefits as well. SAM-e has been used for years in Europe to treat depression, and it definitely shows promise. Still, no large U.S.-based studies have been done to confirm its effectiveness and safety.

SAM-e occurs naturally in your body. It helps spur production of the substances in your brain that regulate mood: dopamine and serotonin. Usually, your body can make all the SAM-e it needs, but depression reduces its levels—hence, the idea to take the compound as a supplement and raise levels back to normal.

You can use SAM-e under medical supervision along with antidepressant drugs or alone for mild-to-moderate depression. For minor depression, the usual dosage is 400 milligrams a day, but you can safely use up to 1,600 milligrams a day, advises Richard Brown, M.D., associate professor of clinical psychiatry at Columbia University in New York City and author of *Stop Depression Now*. The supplement should be taken first thing in the morning, on an empty stomach.

People who have bipolar disorder should not use SAM-e without medical supervision, since any kind of antidepressant can tip them over into a state of mania, cautions Dr. Brown.

You'll want the pills to be enteric-coated to protect your stomach from irritation by preventing them from dissolving until they reach your small intestine. A few good brands suggested by Dr. Brown are Nature Made (by Pharmavite), Puritan Pride, and General Nutrition Center products.

SAM-e has a better chance of working well if you're getting adequate amounts of folate and vitamins B_{12} and B_6 to help it along. Aim for 800 micrograms of folic acid (the synthetic form of folate), 1,000 micrograms of vitamin B_{12}, and 100 milligrams of vitamin B_6, recommends Dr. Brown.

simulating light boxes are also available, but it's best to use these under medical supervision. You may also require more sleep during winter months, as there is some evidence that people who sleep longer have fewer SAD-related symptoms.

Schedule sleep. Irregular sleep/wake cycles can contribute to the symptoms of depression, Dr. Leibenluft says. So keep yours regular by going to bed at the same time every night and getting up at the same time every morning. The more regular your sleep pattern, the more solid your sleep will be. You especially don't want to go to bed so late at night that you sleep through the bright light of morning. Another reason exercise may be very helpful for depression is that it promotes sound sleep.

Get hubby to help with the housework. Sociologist Chloe Bird, Ph.D., of Brown University has found that the larger a woman's share of household chores is, the more likely she is to feel psychologically depressed, especially if she's employed outside the home.

"Housework is less likely to feel like drudgery and is more highly valued by both partners when it's shared," Dr. Bird says. She suggests that couples divide domestic chores evenly. Ideally, each partner should do slightly less than half. Those women who felt least gloomy handled no more than 46 percent. So give yourself a gift by having a third household member or a maid service do the remaining chores.

Protect Your Air Force: Respiratory Health

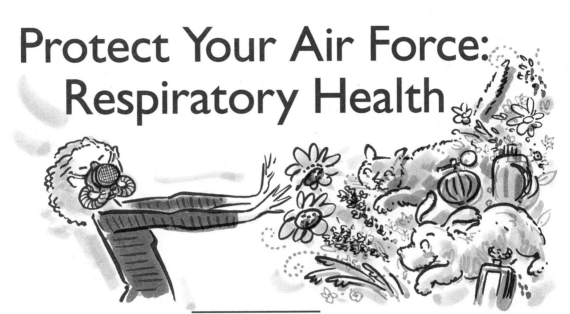

Breathe in, breathe out. Breathe in, breathe out.

For most of us, this basic bodily function doesn't take any conscious thought. But some 17 million Americans with asthma *do* have to think about it because a sudden asthma attack can cause wheezing, coughing, chest tightness . . . and on occasion, an inability to breathe at all. The disease kills more than 5,400 Americans each year.

It works like this: A trigger in the environment—often an allergen such as pollen, dust mites, or a viral infection—invades your bronchial tubes, which move air in and out of your body, and causes inflammation. The surrounding muscles then tighten, and your tubes fill with mucus, making breathing more difficult.

Asthma is another one of those diseases that seems to have a gender bias. It sends women to the emergency room nearly twice as often as men. But we don't have to become its victims. This chronic threat to our air force can be held off, stopped in its tracks, and even pushed back with today's arsenal of therapies.

Risk Factors

Even though environmental factors and allergens appear to affect the course of asthma, we're still not sure exactly what their role is. "We know that viruses and allergen exposure can exacerbate the disease, but we don't really know if they cause it," says Rebecca S. Gruchalla, M.D., Ph.D., chief of the allergy and immunology division at the University of Texas Southwestern Medical Center at Dallas.

For the time being, however, the generally accepted list of risk factors for asthma attacks comprises genetic, environmental, hormonal, allergenic, infectious, climatic, and physiological triggers. Marianne Frieri, M.D., Ph.D., director of allergy immunology training at Nassau County Medical Center/North Shore University Hospital in East Meadow, New York, and associate professor of medicine at the State University of New York in Stony Brook, details them in this way.

Hormones. Our regular hormonal shifts that occur around menstruation and pregnancy, possibly hormone-replacement therapy for postmenopausal women, can trigger asthma.

Occupations. Nurses, teachers, day care–center workers—these largely female workforces report significant problems in their workplaces. These include latex allergies among nurses and, among all of these workers, viral infections from patients and students and reactions to animal dander on clothes and to dust.

Irritants. Plant pollens, mold, fungi, tobacco smoke, wood smoke, air pollution, chemical fumes, strong odors (including perfume), and sprays all can stimulate airways to tighten and clog. Parental smoking is especially harmful to children with asthma, according to one Canadian study. After following a group of children for 6 years, researchers found that those who still had asthma were almost four times as likely to have mothers who smoked heavily as were kids whose symptoms had disappeared.

Animal dander. The dander (not fur) and saliva of cats and the dander of dogs can trigger an asthma attack.

Cockroaches. Allergies to cockroaches pose risks for inner-city residents, especially.

Dust mites. In pillows, mattresses, carpets, and stuffed toys, our airways—not our eyes—detect the droppings of these tiny visitors.

Respiratory infections. Colds and the flu may bring on asthma troubles.

Exercise. Exercise-induced asthma is very common and controllable with medication. Research suggests that drinking water before, during, and after workouts is important for women with asthma. Women with the disease may start out with a hydration deficit that could make their asthma worse.

Cold, dry air. As some runners and skiers will tell you, breathing cold, dry air can launch an asthma attack.

Drugs. Aspirin, ibuprofen, and other non-steroidal anti-inflammatory drugs (NSAIDs) are also offenders.

Anxiety. Stress and worry alone may not provoke an attack but may contribute to one.

Foods. Children in particular can be sensitive to milk, eggs, peanuts, nuts, soy, wheat, and fish. Sensitivity to shellfish is more common in adults.

Allergic rhinitis. Also known as hay fever, this condition is a red flag, too. It afflicts more than three-quarters of all people with asthma.

Prevention

Avoiding trouble in the first place is a big part of asthma prevention. Stay away from triggers and allergens that can spark an attack. If that isn't practical, allergy shots, or "immunotherapy," can make you less sensitive.

The next line of defense is early detection. "When it starts out, asthma is completely reversible," says Martha V. White, M.D., research director of the Institute for Asthma and Allergy at Washington Hospital Center in Washington, D.C. But once inflammation of the airways takes hold, the damage can be permanent. The lungs develop scar tissue that sometimes can't be reversed. Still, even at that point, proper monitoring can help keep attacks under control.

"What most people don't know about asthma is that it's really, really controllable," says Dr. White. But asthma can range from mild to life-threatening, so it's important to know where your symptoms fall. That's where a device called a peak flow meter comes in.

Basically, it's a little tube you blow into twice daily that tells you how open or closed your large airways are. Because asthma rarely flares up without warning signs that appear hours beforehand, the meter works like an "asthma thermometer," Dr. White says, to detect trouble before it escalates.

Medications are a regular part of life for

many women with asthma. Those with the mildest form of the disease often are prescribed quick-relief, or "rescue," medications alone. These are bronchodilators taken with inhalers as needed. They work within about 10 minutes to open the airways. For more severe asthma, anti-inflammatory medicines called controller medications are used regularly to keep symptoms reined in. Most of these drugs, which include steroids, are also delivered to the lungs via inhalers.

Except for those with very mild asthma, most people require treatment with both types of medications, according to Dr. White. Taking medicine as prescribed is key to managing this disease, but not everyone follows that advice.

"People often think that controller medications should work right away, but these anti-inflammatories take awhile," relates Dr. White. "It's like taking an antibiotic: It takes a day or two before it kicks in." Those who think that their medication doesn't work fast enough tend to rely on rescue medication alone, leaving them more vulnerable to attacks.

Here are Dr. White's tips for breathing easier with (and without) an inhaler.

Try an instant inhaler substitute. Stuck without your bronchodilator and feel an attack coming on? Grab a cup of coffee or caffeinated cola, says Dr. White. Caffeine is very similar chemically to one of the rescue medications.

EMPHYSEMA

Would you rather (a) die prematurely, (b) spend the rest of your life tethered to an oxygen tank, (c) develop a barrel chest, or (d) grunt every time you let out a breath? This multiple choice comes with a bleak bonus: If you have emphysema, you can pick all four.

As the most common cause of respiratory disease death in the United States, emphysema is tragic because it's almost entirely preventable. Up to 90 percent of cases can be blamed on smoking. (The rest are due to inherited gene deficiency). It takes its time, too: "Emphysema can be a long, slow decline," says Monica Kraft, M.D., a pulmonologist and assistant professor of medicine at the National Jewish Medical and Research Center in Denver.

The word itself describes the disease. Its Greek root means "to inflate," and that's the problem: Lungs overinflate because of inefficient breathing. With emphysema, the air sacs in the lungs become overstretched or break. This makes your lungs less elastic, so air is trapped in your chest and you have to work harder to breathe (hence, the barrel chest and grunting on exhale).

In most of the two-million-plus Americans with emphysema, the disease has been doing its dirty work for years before it's diagnosed. The first symptom is often shortness of breath. Eventually, supplementary oxygen or even a lung transplant may be needed.

While emphysema prefers men by a margin of more than 50 percent, women are catching up.

There's some silver lining to this cloud of smoking disease. "It's never too late to quit smoking," assures Dr. Kraft. "We know that patients who smoke have an accelerated decline in lung function," she reports, but shortly after becoming smoke-free, an ex-smoker's rate of decline reaches that of a person who never smoked.

Tap liquid relief. If you're minus both your inhaler and a caffeinated beverage, drink hot water. Dr. White says that it can soothe the chest.

Work the phone. If an attack hits while you're away from home and you can get to a phone and a drugstore, call your doctor and have her call in your inhaler prescription so you can pick it up at the pharmacy. Depending on the distance, it may be faster and safer than trying to reach your inhaler at home.

Steer clear of car storage. Extreme heat and cold can ruin inhalers, so don't stash yours in your car.

Any way that you can change your environment to minimize exposure to triggers is one more way to keep asthma from controlling your life. Allergy and asthma experts recommend these breath-saving strategies for common home-front triggers.

Freshen that fur. Bathe your pet (or have someone else do it) once a week to minimize dander.

Get into hot water. Wash all bedding (including pillows), clothes, and stuffed toys in hot water at least once a week to control dust mites. Investing in mite covers may help as well.

Clean the carpet weekly. Dust mites love that sheared plush even more than you do.

Cut wet-air woes. Use a dehumidifier to dry out damp basements and bathrooms, favorite haunts of molds and fungi.

Ban the bugs. Get rid of cockroaches with boric acid and traps.

Hang out with the healthy. Avoid contact with people who have colds or the flu to reduce your chances of infection.

Clear the air. Don't smoke, and don't allow it in your home.

Making breathing easier when you're away from home can be a challenge. Try these tips for travel comfort.

REAL-LIFE SCENARIO

Her Bronchitis Just Won't Go Away

Anna, 43, has been running a day care center out of her home for years, and she's had great luck not only in her business but also with her health. Unlike the assistant providers she has hired, she has never fallen prey to the many colds and flu viruses that the kids bring with them to the center. But this year has been different. Although she has never smoked, gets plenty of rest and exercise, and takes lots of vitamin C, she has come down with a cold that just won't go away. It started as a scratchy throat, then quickly went to her chest. Now, 8 weeks later, she sometimes coughs hard, brings up mucus, and is short of breath. Her doctor had her lungs x-rayed, but there is no sign of disease. What should she do?

Anna may not have bronchitis at all. This word gets used very broadly to describe a number of respiratory ailments, but the coughing and mucus could be caused by something else.

As a day care worker, she's certainly exposed to lots of different viruses from the children at her center. She has probably developed an upper respiratory infection from one such virus, and the result is what we call twitchy, or reactive, airways. This means that the bronchial tubes that supply her lungs with air have become more responsive to various stimuli, including allergens, irritants, and viruses. As a result, the airways may have narrowed and become inflamed, leading to her coughing and shortness of breath.

In with the good air, out with the bad. Before starting a long car trip, turn on the air conditioner or heater and open the windows for 10 minutes before climbing in. This helps remove dust mites and molds that lurk in the ventilating system, carpets, and upholstery.

Time your travel. Steer clear of car travel when pollution is heaviest in the daytime. Air quality is better in the early morning and late evening.

Get "flight insurance." On international flights that allow smoking, request a seat as far

Another strong possibility is that Anna has an underlying element of asthma brought on only by viral infection. We know that, like cold air, smoke, strong odors, or allergens such as ragweed, viral infection is one of the triggers that can bring on an asthma attack. Note that she's coughing and not wheezing: There is a syndrome called cough-variant asthma where people exhibit only coughing, as opposed to the classic wheezing of asthma.

The mucus that Anna is coughing up needs examining: if it's clear, that points to a viral infection that's producing twitchy airways. If it's green, she may have a bacterial infection on top of a possible allergy, and I'd probably put her on an antibiotic. If she has asthma and is coughing up yellow mucus, the problem may be an allergy rather than infection. The only way to tell is with a microscope, so I'd get a sample and examine the cells.

Anna should consult with either an asthma or allergy specialist to pinpoint just what's causing her symptoms, and then take appropriate action. If it turns out that she does have asthma, she may be able to stop it from becoming worse and to reverse her breathing problems.

Expert consulted
Rebecca S. Gruchalla, M.D., Ph.D.
Chief of the allergy and immunology division
University of Texas Southwestern Medical
*   Center*
Dallas

as possible from the puffers. If your asthma is sometimes severe enough to require additional oxygen, you may feel the need at 35,000 feet. Make arrangements with the airline well in advance for supplemental oxygen.

Pack it in. When you travel, keep your inhaler in your purse or carry-on—not in checked baggage that is out of your reach and can go astray.

Be a picky eater. If you have an asthma reaction to certain foods, be wary of in-flight meals. No one on board will know what's in those premade dishes, so if you can, eat at home and take some snacks with you on the plane.

Signs and Symptoms

The warning signs of asthma can vary from person to person, and from attack to attack. If you've already been diagnosed with asthma, a drop in the peak flow reading is a sure sign of an attack. Here are some of the other most common symptoms: labored breathing or wheezing; chronic cough, especially at night; fast breathing; shortness of breath; and chest tightness or discomfort. Symptoms of allergic rhinitis, such as fatigue, a scratchy throat, headache, head congestion, or itchy, watery eyes, often occur along with asthma flare-ups.

Don't Panic!

Some fairly minor conditions can make you wrongly suspect that asthma is filching your air. Dr. White mentions these.

Indigestion. It can bring on the tight-chest feeling that marks asthma.

Sinus infections. You can't breathe freely, so these painful pretenders can be misinterpreted.

Nasal congestion. Trying to breathe through a blocked-up, stuffy nose is like trying to suck a milkshake through a wet paper straw, notes Dr. White. Open your mouth to make breathing easier.

Bronchitis. Its coughing, wheezing, and chest tightness can closely mimic asthma.

"The bottom line is, if you're having chest discomfort and trouble breathing, have it checked out," advises Dr. White.

Who Do I See?

A primary-care physician is often the first and only professional consulted. If a specialist is needed, it's usually an allergist/immunologist or a pulmonologist (lung doctor). If you think you have the symptoms of asthma, you should seek treatment, says Dr. Frieri. Postponing care is dangerous; permanent harm may be done to your lungs.

Unlike time-pressed general practitioners, a specialist can take 40 minutes or more to obtain a detailed personal history, says Dr. Frieri. "When giving your personal history, you need to focus on all the factors that may be contributing to asthma: the environment at work and home, the presence of cats or dogs, what a woman uses for cleaning, whether or not she has kids, and so on. Then there are conditions like hay fever, ear infections, and sinusitis. Does she sneeze, wheeze, or cough? And what's the family history of respiratory problems with parents and grandparents?"

What Can I Expect?

During a physical exam, the doctor will concentrate on the upper and lower airways, looking into your ears, nose, and throat and listening to your chest for any signs of wheezing. This may be followed by a pulmonary function test called spirometry: you breathe into a calibrated instrument that measures things like your lung capacity and how much air you exhale in 1 second. This detects any obstruction or restriction in your breathing.

WOMEN ASK WHY

Why do some women go back to smoking years after giving it up?

Weight is the critical reason that many women, particularly those going through menopause, resume smoking after years of being smoke-free. When we talk to women who have quit smoking and then relapse, that's the most important factor that they cite.

Women and girls learn early on that smoking instead of eating is a method of controlling weight. It's true that smokers on average weigh less than nonsmokers, and when menopausal women experience the weight gain that can be common with this stage of life, some do turn back to cigarettes.

There's another factor at work here, though. We have a growing body of knowledge that indicates that the ability to resist smoking or any addiction is related to a sense of empowerment. What's interesting is how this is reflected in the field of medicine: Fewer than 5 percent of physicians now smoke. Although nurses are quitting smoking, too, or taking it up in smaller numbers, there's a big gap in their ranks: Licensed practical nurses (L.P.N.'s) have about 1½ times the

You may also get a chest x-ray to pinpoint an abnormality in your lungs or take an allergy test to find out what substances are triggering allergic reactions.

Emotional as well as physical reactions can be a real issue for women with asthma. "When you have asthma, it feels like you're suffocating," notes Dorothea Lack, Ph.D., clinical assistant professor in the psychiatry department at the University of California, San Francisco. "The memory of a past attack sets up an anticipatory anxiety that can snowball into a new attack," she observes. And in the midst of that attack, the fear of imminent death is overwhelming.

Those anxious feelings can be among a

smoking rate of registered nurses. And L.P.N.'s have less formal education and tend to make less money.

This smoking "gap" mirrors the overall relationship between income, power, and smoking, regardless of gender. The lower someone's socioeconomic status, the higher their smoking risk.

Many women also use smoking as a reward. They work at a paying job all day, sometimes two jobs, then go home and work all evening. Smoking presents a time-out or respite from those demands. The cigarette industry capitalizes on this with ads that show a powerful image: a woman in a garden . . . alone . . . being still . . . smoking.

Overall, the incidence of women smokers 18 and older is declining. But for females under 18, the numbers are going up. So what we're seeing is a transient dip in smoking among grown-up women, which will be more than made up for by the next generation.

Expert consulted
Barbara A. Phillips, M.D.
Professor of pulmonary and critical-care medi-
cine
University of Kentucky Medical Center
Lexington

asthma," reports Dr. Lack. "That's when you see if their medication can be adjusted, and you start them on relaxation training."

Since you can't be deeply relaxed and anxious at the same time, she recommends these keys for calming down during an asthma attack.

Listen and learn. With commercially available relaxation tapes, you can learn to use imagery to quiet the panicky feelings that contribute to an asthma episode.

Practice, practice. Listen to relaxation tapes once a day for 30 days to practice techniques like visualizing, tensing and relaxing your muscles, and deep breathing.

Maintain for a month. Practice relaxation techniques daily for a month, advises Dr. Lack, and you'll be able to practice less often and still call up the relaxation response when needed. "You won't get instant results, so stick with it," she urges.

woman's biggest challenges with asthma because of their circular link with the disease, according to Dr. Lack. An attack can trigger panic, panic can make the attack worse, and round and round it goes.

Adding to the tension, asthma medicines can cause anxiety-like side effects. Dr. White's own study of more than 1,800 people with asthma showed that roughly 60 percent experienced various side effects from their medication, including shakiness and jitteriness. As a result, up to one-third of adults skipped or reduced doses.

"Often, a patient will come in appearing to have an anxiety disorder, and then you find out that they're taking a bronchodilator for their

Conventional Wisdom

While there is no cure for asthma, the closest thing is good old allergy shots, says Dr. White—assuming the asthma is mostly related to an allergy. The goal is to lower your number of triggers. "The more triggers you can eliminate, the better you can tolerate the ones you still have," she says.

Allergy shots work like vaccinations: You're injected with the substance that provokes the problem, in small, increasing doses over several months. Maintenance doses can then continue for several years. As you build immunity to the trigger allergen, you substantially reduce your misery.

While controller and rescue drugs are effective at quieting inflammation and opening airways after the fact, they may be replaced in the future by medicines that prevent the problem in the first place. Today, inhaled steroids of several types (though steroids can also be taken in pill or liquid form) are the main defense in controlling inflammation. And for acute attacks, bronchodilators in several different classes all ease the muscles around airways so that normal breathing can resume. Among the newer entries are leukotriene inhibitors.

What's coming up? A nonspecific allergy shot called anti-IgE could conceivably control all allergies and asthma by suppressing the allergic reaction. It's been "far more effective in asthma control than I ever imagined," in clinical trials, reports Dr. White. It's a few years away from introduction, though. Also exciting and in development are two drugs that would interrupt the inflammation process even earlier than anti-IgE.

In the meantime, however, experts advise that you follow your doctor's instructions closely and work with your physician to stay on top of your needs. "Asthma therapy is a very fluid thing. You don't just go on medication and stay there for a year," explains Dr. White. If you can anticipate flare-ups, such as just before a menstrual period or when you know you'll be outside during a high-pollen time, talk with your doctor about temporarily boosting your controller medication, she suggests.

"The people who don't pay attention

AN OLD ENEMY RETURNS: TUBERCULOSIS

We don't think about tuberculosis much anymore. It's a disease we'd thought we'd conquered—until recently.

After 1953, when national surveillance of tuberculosis (TB) began, the number of reported cases steadily decreased. Yet, starting in 1985, the incidence of the disease began to increase and peaked in 1992. Experts think that this may have happened as a result of the AIDS epidemic, which has left so many people with suppressed immune systems. Fortunately, improved TB-control programs have again put the disease on the decline. There were only 18,361 cases in 1998—the lowest rate since 1953.

Tuberculosis is an airborne infection, which means it can be spread through coughing, sneezing, laughing, or even singing. But you would need prolonged exposure to an infected person before you came down with the disease. It usually attacks the lungs, but it can also affect other organs and tissues.

The symptoms of TB range from prolonged coughing, including coughing up blood; fever; chills or night sweats; lethargy; weakness; unexplained weight loss; or loss of appetite. People at higher risk for contracting the disease are those who, like teachers, health-care workers, and prison guards, interact with infected persons or high-risk populations; the poor and medically underserved; people with suppressed immune systems; and the elderly. If you have reason to think that you may have been exposed to TB or are experiencing TB symptoms, see your doctor immediately because, untreated, it can spread to others.

To detect tuberculosis, doctors use either a Mantoux skin test, in which a small amount of tuberculin is injected into the top layers of skin on the forearm, or a tuberculin tine test, a skin test using multiple punctures that contain the testing material. The results are obvious 2 to 3 days after the test, with definite raised bumps on the skin an indication of positive results. Your doctor may also order chest x-rays and sputum tests.

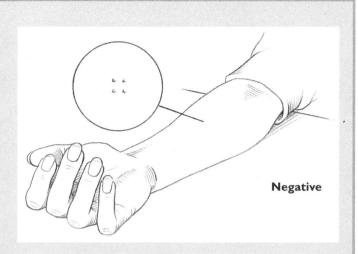

Negative

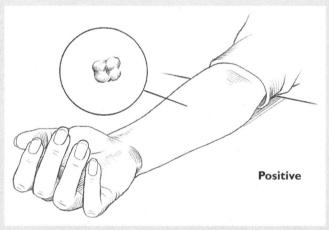

Positive

If your test comes back positive, it doesn't mean an end to daily life as you know it. Most TB, more than 90 percent, can be cured with medications, but they have to be taken regularly for 6 months and often longer. Newly approved drugs combine the three main medications into one pill or require less frequent doses.

Incorrectly or incompletely treated, however, TB could progress into multidrug resistant tuberculosis (MDR TB), which does not respond to two or more of the primary treatment drugs, and this resistance spreads with the disease. Response rates of MDR TB plummet to less than 50 percent.

to their symptoms," warns Dr. Gruchalla, "are the ones who can end up in the emergency room."

Great Alternatives

"You can chase asthma symptoms forever, but the key is to treat the causes," says Beverly Yates, N.D., a naturopathic physician practicing in Seattle. While supporting the benefits of steroid medications to handle severe attacks, she reports that reliance on natural medicine can lessen—sometimes even erase—the need for inhalers and pills. Work with your doctor to find alternatives that are right for you.

These supplement and herb strategies get the nod from Dr. Yates to help lessen the impact of asthma.

Get fat(ty). Expand your intake of omega-3 fatty acids by eating cold-water fish like salmon and mackerel, extra virgin olive oil, sunflower seeds, and pumpkin seeds. Dr. Yates recommends a five-to-one balance of omega-6 fatty acids (as found in red meat) to omega-3's. She suggests eating these foods at least once a week, and preferably three to five times a week. But if you decide to stick with supplements, aim for 200 milligrams of omega-3, she advises, and maintain your regular diet. (If you eat an average Western diet, you're probably getting enough omega-6's.)

Keep going with ginkgo. This Asian leaf helps block constriction in the bronchial tubes. About 200 milligrams per day is recommended. As with any herb, don't expect immediate improvement. "Herbs, as medicinal foods, take time," says Dr. Yates. "I usually say to patients, 'Give me a month for every year you've had the problem to see results.'" She recommends, however, taking a holiday from supplements—a week off for every week on. Do not use with antidepressant MAO-inhibitor drugs, aspirin or other nonsteroidal anti-inflammatory medications, or blood-thinning medications.

Breathe easier with evening primrose. Especially for women whose symptoms flare up just before their periods, Dr. Yates recommends taking 1 teaspoon of evening primrose oil twice daily during the premenstrual week to reduce airway inflammation. As an alternative, Dr. Yates suggests taking 1,500 to 3,000 milligrams of evening primrose oil capsules, divided up throughout the day, with food.

Magnify magnesium. Calcium can be aggravating for some people with asthma, reports Dr. Yates, and these same people are often low in magnesium, which may help relax the smooth muscle of airways. Up to 400 milligrams a day can be helpful, she says, but if you have heart or kidney problems, check with your doctor before

taking magnesium doses of more than 350 milligrams. Also, magnesium may cause diarrhea in some people.

Calm with coleus forskohlii. There's some evidence that this herb may be as effective at quieting inflammation as some prescription asthma drugs, without jittery side effects. The usual dose is 50 milligrams two or three times a day. Because it may enhance the effects of medications for asthma or high blood pressure, with negative results, do *not* use coleus forskohlii without medical supervision, and always talk with your doctor before adjusting your asthma prescriptions.

Dr. Yates also advocates two other measures to keep air flowing freely: massage and yoga.

Massage. The chest and upper respiratory cavity can benefit from massage because it helps the body clear out waste products that asthma helps build.

Power breathing. Yoga's breathing exercises are a terrific tool, avows Dr. Yates. "If an attack is stress-related, you could use your breath to calm things down before trouble starts."

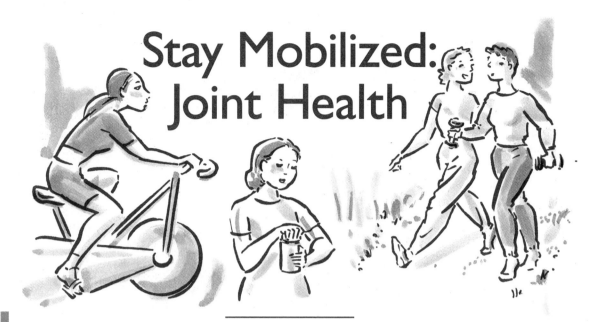

Stay Mobilized: Joint Health

It's not a new problem. Even the dinosaurs had it. But despite its reputation as an affliction of the elderly, arthritis—the catchall term for almost 100 diseases—plays no favorites when it comes to age. Kids, teenagers, and young adults are fair game, too.

The word itself means inflammation or damage to joints, but some varieties of the disease can extend to muscles, skin, and organs. And since women are the favored targets for many forms of this sometimes debilitating condition, new treatment and prevention tools are especially good news for us. "I've worked in arthritis research for more than 16 years, and things are changing," says Leigh F. Callahan, Ph.D., associate director of the Thurston Arthritis Research Center at the University of North Carolina at Chapel Hill. "There's a good feeling about where we are now in treating arthritis."

"We don't see as many wheelchairs in our clinics as in the past," confirms Melanie J. Harrison, M.D., attending rheumatologist at the Hospital for Special Surgery in New York City. "Fewer people are coming in with contracted hands and destroyed fingers."

The reason is that potent new drugs with fewer side effects exist these days. And there is mounting evidence that moderate exercise helps people with arthritis, who currently number some one in six Americans. In addition, acupuncture is gaining ground in pain relief, while naturopathic doctors are using supplements like glucosamine sulfate with good results. More than ever before, when a woman is told that she has arthritis, it isn't the end of active living, but the start of an action plan.

Risk Factors

Despite its variety of forms and names (osteoarthritis, rheumatoid arthritis, gout, and many others), the one thing we don't know about arthritis is what causes it. And that makes pinpointing risk factors iffy.

"We know that some forms are related to genetics. Osteoarthritis is linked to overuse and abuse. And bacteria may be triggers for some forms in some people," explains Teresa J. Brady, Ph.D., medical advisor to the Arthritis Foundation in Atlanta. "We are certain, though, that it's definitely not an inevitable part of aging."

Most common is osteoarthritis, the wear-and-tear form. Cushioning joint cartilage breaks down, causing bone to bump against bone in specific places like your hands, knees, hips, feet, and back. Rheumatoid arthritis, a whole-body autoimmune disease, takes a different toll. Your body's natural immune system attacks its own healthy joint tissue, causing swelling and damage. Following are the factors that can increase risk.

Gender. Some 74 percent of all osteoarthritis, or 15.3 million cases, occurs in women. Rheumatoid arthritis prefers women, too—we're about 1.5 million, or 71 percent of U.S. cases.

Family ties. Genetics plays a role, especially in rheumatoid arthritis, where a primary risk is having a parent or sibling with the disease, relates Dr. Harrison.

Age. While arthritis strikes all ages, osteoarthritis predominantly targets those over 45.

History of joint damage. Whether it's a tear in a knee ligament that happened while you were skiing, an inflammation, or a repetitive hand motion, injury or chronic strain on a joint can increase your risk of osteoarthritis.

Overweight. Are you overweight, 45 or older, and of average height? Research shows that if you lost 11 pounds or more over 10 years, you would cut your risk for developing osteoarthritis of the knee in half.

Inactivity. There's evidence that exercise not only helps reduce pain but also lessens wear and tear on joints by keeping surrounding muscles strong.

WOMEN ASK WHY

Why is carpal tunnel syndrome everywhere today though it was unheard of 20 years ago?

Twenty years ago, we didn't have a lot of people typing on computer keyboards.

Carpal tunnel syndrome (CTS) is often associated with chronic, repetitive motion of the hands and wrists combined with excessive force. This combination compresses the nerve that supplies feeling to the palm side of the thumb and first two fingers. This nerve passes from your arm to your hand right beneath the carpal ligament, which is part of the carpal tunnel, or canal. The result of nerve compression can be numbness and shooting pain.

So what does all this have to do with computer keyboards? These days, many workers are practically tethered to their computers, sitting for hours at a time. Rather than distributing physical forces across many muscle groups, they're making the same typing motions and using a mouse over and over again—and with too much force. They also don't keep their wrists straight, and they hold their arms in the "action-ready" position even when not typing—all in all, a recipe for trouble.

But computer use is only part of the answer. The other part is the *appearance* of growth in the number of CTS cases because of advances in diagnosis. Better techniques for detecting nerve problems now help correctly identify cases of CTS that before that time may have been blamed on something like insufficient blood supply.

These steps can help alleviate CTS.

Prevention

You don't have to sit and wait to become a statistic in America's leading cause of disability. Here's how you can avoid or reduce the impact of arthritis.

Get a head start. Joint damage can be slowed down and even prevented in some cases

Be wristwise. A keyboard wrist support isn't a leaning post. Let your hands float over it, like a pianist's, while you type.

Lead with your left. If you're right-handed, you're better off manipulating a computer mouse with your left hand (and vice versa). It eases strain by resting your dominant hand and, for righties, by eliminating the reach to get around the number keypad on the right side of the keyboard.

Perfect your posture. Keep your upper back in contact with your chair to prevent the rounded, hunched shoulders that can result in tighter pectoral muscles. When these muscles tighten, they may compress vessels and nerves as they enter the arm.

Take time-outs. When you're not working the keys, put your hands in your lap or let them hang at your sides to rest muscles and nerves.

Try a trackball. It requires less clutching action than a mouse and lets your hand stay open and more relaxed.

Go with cruise control. When cruising the Internet, move your mouse pad and mouse to your lap and lean back slightly in your chair. This reduces stress on your back, shoulder, wrist, and fingers.

Expert consulted
Margit L. Bleecker, M.D., Ph.D.
Director
Center for Occupational and Environmental
*   Neurology*
Baltimore

Find the facts. Because treatment can vary dramatically for different types of arthritis, it's important to know what kind you may have, advises Dr. Lee.

Maintain a fighting weight. You can fight off osteoarthritis by lightening the load on your weight-bearing knees and hips. Being overweight has a domino effect, Dr. Callahan notes. It promotes inactivity, leading to limited joint movement, which fosters joint stiffening.

Get up, get out, get moving. Daily exercise keeps joints flexible, dampens pain, and tones up joint-supporting muscles. If Dr. Brady had osteoarthritis, she would start an exercise plan that would keep her active without aggravating joint pain—such as a plan that includes swimming, walking, or riding a stationary bicycle. But before starting any kind of exercise regimen, work with your doctor to figure out what is right for you.

Feed your health. Experts counsel that a balanced diet helps maintain weight and nourish joints, muscles, and bones. There's evidence that omega-3 fatty acids, the kind found in salmon, anchovies, mackerel, tuna, and sardines, may lower the risk of rheumatoid arthritis.

"C" the light. Vitamin C may help slow down osteoarthritis of the knee, according to one study. Those who ate the most C had less pain and cartilage loss than those eating the least (120 milligrams, or about two medium-size oranges per day).

Read for relief. Go to school—"Arthritis School." The Arthritis Foundation has a self-help course available in most states to help you eat right and manage pain, among other things. One

if you get diagnosed and treated early. "Don't listen to old wives' tales about arthritis," cautions Sicy H. Lee, M.D., assistant clinical professor of medicine at New York University School of Medicine and attending physician at the Hospital for Joint Diseases, both in New York City. "Lots of people think that there's nothing you can do about arthritis, and that isn't so."

WOMEN ASK WHY

Why do joints crack and creak more as people get older?

Inside your joints, wear and tear of cartilage, ligaments, and bones occur as they rub against each other over the years. If your neck cracks when you move it a certain way or your knees crack when you go up or down stairs, it may not be any cause for concern. When a patient says to me, "My knees crack. Do I have to worry about it?" I say, "If it doesn't bother you, no. Don't worry."

If cracking noises are accompanied by other symptoms, such as painful movement, however, it could be a sign of osteoarthritis. Let's say that a doctor examines those cracking knees. When she moves the knees a certain way, you have pain. When she examines your kneecaps, she can feel crepitans, which are the loose bits of cartilage that can cause creaking. And along with that, you have pain when climbing stairs. All these symptoms together could point to early osteoarthritis. If you complain, "My neck cracks," and it doesn't hurt and you have full range of movement, a doctor might just respond by telling you, "Stop cracking it—don't push it." But general cracking and creaking, especially in a younger person, don't have much significance.

Expert consulted
Sicy H. Lee, M.D.
Assistant clinical professor of medicine
New York University School of Medicine
New York City

beware the complaint that lingers. See your doctor if any of these symptoms in or around a joint persists for more than 2 weeks: pain, stiffness, swelling, and trouble moving a joint.

One of the biggest differences between the two most common forms of arthritis is the kind of swelling that occurs, says Dr. Harrison. "In rheumatoid arthritis, you get a soft swelling—it squooshes, unlike osteoarthritis, where you get bony swelling," says the rheumatologist. Other rheumatoid arthritis cues are a whole-body morning stiffness, flulike fatigue, fever, and decreased appetite.

Don't Panic!

Not every achy elbow means arthritis, of course. Because the disease takes so many forms, you could have one of the lesser-known types of arthritis. What else might stiffness or fever mean?

Bursitis or tendinitis, both temporary inflammatory joint conditions, says Dr. Brady, can appear like osteoarthritis. They can surface suddenly and stop within days or weeks.

Arthritis-like symptoms very similar to rheumatoid arthritis can also be caused by viruses, according to Dr. Harrison. Two common suspects are parvovirus B19, with feverish symptoms often passed from school-age children to young mothers, and hepatitis C, which can swell the small joints of the hands. The various aches and pains of common flu viruses can also be mistaken for arthritis.

The finger tingling and numbness that come with carpal tunnel syndrome can be associated

study of the 6-week course found that it pared pain by 18 percent and saved hundreds of dollars on doctor visits. For information, call the Foundation's National Information Hotline at (800) 283-7800.

Signs and Symptoms

An errant golf swing or a misstep on the stairs can cause temporary woe to a wrist or knee, but

with rheumatoid arthritis, but they can also be unrelated to any medical condition.

Who Do I See?

Your primary-care physician is the one to start and possibly stay with, advises Dr. Brady, as long as she is current on developments in the disease. While an arthritis specialist like a rheumatologist or an endocrinologist isn't necessarily the next step, she says, "You absolutely need someone who stays up-to-date. If your physician says, 'Oh, it's just arthritis, learn to live with it,' that's your cue to get another opinion."

For exercise to ease or reduce symptoms, you may get a referral to see a physical therapist or an occupational therapist.

Seeking out another opinion from an expert in alternative medicine is an option that even the federal government seems eager to explore these days. Dr. Callahan has been involved with a study for the National Institutes of Health, exploring alternative options in arthritis treatment. "We queried physicians and found that 49 percent would recommend some form of alternative therapies," she reports.

What Can I Expect?

Because there is no arthritis cure, treatment focuses on managing the condition. "An appropriate management plan needs to go beyond medications, which are the first things people think about," observes Dr.

RHEUMATOID ARTHRITIS

Many patients of Melanie J. Harrison, M.D., are looking and feeling better these days and spending less time in the hospital. The reason is that "new drugs and other therapies have changed the symptoms and course of rheumatoid arthritis we see in our clinics," says the attending rheumatologist at the Hospital for Special Surgery in New York City.

This change for the better is especially welcome because of the seriousness of rheumatoid arthritis (RA). "RA is a rapidly progressive disease that can be very crippling over a short amount of time," says Dr. Harrison. And it strikes women up to three times more often than men. Unlike osteoarthritis, which affects joints only, RA is a systemic disease that invades the entire body.

For reasons yet unknown, the natural immune system of a woman with RA starts attacking her body's own healthy joint tissue. Symptoms include fatigue, stiffness (especially in the morning), joint swelling and redness, and lumps under the skin, called nodules. The resulting inflammation and joint damage can lead to severe deformity. Life expectancy can shrink by 3 years in women with RA, and half of RA sufferers can't work within 10 years after the condition starts.

This gloomy picture is brightening, though. "Don't think for a minute that a diagnosis of RA is a sentence," avows Dr. Harrison, a rheumatologist and medical advisor to the Arthritis Foundation in Atlanta. "We have new drugs that seem to alter the course of the disease and a lot of additional treatments that can help with symptoms." The drugs are DMARDs (disease-modifying antirheumatic drugs) that reduce the inflammation and seem to slow the advance of RA—possibly even stop it in its tracks.

"They address the serious effects of RA, such as muscle wasting and joint contraction from disuse," says Dr. Harrison. Physical and occupational therapy techniques, especially aquatic exercises, are effective in strengthening muscles and promoting mobility, she notes.

What's more, there are now products available to ease everyday tasks made difficult by swollen, painful joints, such as ergonomically designed devices to help people button and unbutton their shirts.

Brady. "Just as important are self-management strategies, such as losing weight, taking up appropriate physical activity, and trying to take the strain off affected joints."

In addition to these strategies, more common treatments include taking hot baths, using cold packs, protecting joints with braces and splints, and, when necessary, undergoing surgery to replace worn-out joints.

But women with arthritis suffer more than joint pain. They feel the ache of emotional pain as well. "In a very dramatic way, arthritis interrupts your ability to function," says Susan Brace, R.N., Ph.D., a clinical psychologist practicing in Los Angeles. "Little things like cutting with a fork may become impossible. That makes us scared that we might not always be independent."

Dr. Brace recommends the following tactics for handling the psychological impact of arthritis.

Call on your support team. Loved ones need to know that you may be frustrated at not being able to do some things and that this can lead to anger or despair. "It's important to express those feelings and to be heard by people around you," she says.

Come out swinging. "Say, 'I won't be stopped by this.' Don't give up life," urges Dr. Brace. "Arthritis can damage your joints, it's true; but your spirit is made out of something else."

Conventional Wisdom

Medical professionals have made great strides over the past few years in treating arthritis with both drugs and exercise. Here are some of the

WOMAN TO WOMAN

She Uses Yoga to Control Her Arthritis Pain

Like her mother, Lois S. Hazel has osteoarthritis of the spine. But unlike her mother, this 54-year-old publishing professional in Kintnersville, Pennsylvania, is using yoga as a gentle antidote to her symptoms. Her results include more benefits than she bargained for. Here's her story.

When I was in my late forties, my back pain drove me to an orthopedic surgeon. He advised physical activity to strengthen muscles that support the back and to increase flexibility. I needed an outlet from the stressful marketing job I was doing at the time—something to relax me (I have high blood pressure). Yoga seemed like a good way to achieve all those things.

I tried a beginner's Sivananda yoga class at a nearby fitness center and immediately fell in love with it. Like all yoga disciplines, Sivananda puts the emphasis on breathing, relaxation, and correct posture. The stress relief came almost immediately. After the first class, I could have slept like a baby, yet I felt renewed and calm.

It was the most amazing thing I had ever experienced—like a superdrug with no bad side effects. I went back again and again, and I can still say that after 6 years, I've never been disappointed.

Every once in a while, I have a flare-up, which is common

most current weapons they're using to battle the disease.

Cox-2 inhibitors. These quiet both pain and inflammation but with a big difference from previous medications: They don't cause the stomach upset of their cousins, the nonsteroidal anti-inflammatory drugs (NSAIDs).

DMARDs. This abbreviation is short for disease-modifying antirheumatic drugs. Two of these medications, leflunomide (Arava) and cyclosporine (Neoral) are now FDA-approved to put the brakes on rheumatoid arthritis. Cy-

with osteoarthritis. It feels like a giant hand reaching in and squeezing around my spine very, very hard. The pain can literally take my breath away. I will gasp, stop what I'm doing, and do some yoga breathing or at least reposition myself to get relief. I'll find a quiet place to do some yoga stretches, and the improvement is always noticeable.

Yoga has also helped lower my blood pressure, and it was a godsend when I had oral surgery recently. I calmed myself before the surgery with yoga breathing, and that helped me get through the procedure with minimum stress.

I like to do things naturally, so I tried glucosamine sulfate and chondroitin sulfate, which I know work well for many people with arthritis. My brother-in-law, a physical therapist, recommended these supplements to me because they worked wonderfully for some of his patients. After 5 months, I saw no change, really, so I just stayed with yoga, plus walking every day and an occasional over-the-counter pain reliever. To keep my back muscles strong, I also do abdominal exercises.

Taking up yoga was one of the best decisions I ever made about my health. When the pain hits, if I just remember to breathe and concentrate the breath into my spine, it absolutely works. I can literally feel that giant hand softening, relaxing its hold.

My mother was severely debilitated by arthritis in her later years, and I don't want to end up the same way. Yoga is helping me take a different path.

closporin was a drug originally developed to prevent organ rejection in transplant patients. Both actually slow the disease's damage before it becomes irreversible.

Viscosupplements. These substances are replacements for hyaluronic acid, the slippery substance in joint fluid that arthritis takes away. To ease pain in people with mild to moderate osteoarthritis of the knee, viscosupplements are injected directly into the knee joint.

Exercise. "More and more studies show that walking and other kinds of activity can really help people with arthritis," affirms Dr. Callahan. Bicycling, dancing, yoga, and water exercises can all help reduce stiffness and pain.

Great Alternatives

"Glucosamine sulfate can create new cartilage tissue," declares Lorilee Schoenbeck, N.D., a naturopathic physician in Shelburne, Vermont. Citing colleagues who have found x-ray evidence of this phenomenon, Dr. Schoenbeck says that she uses the supplement especially for her patients with affected knees—commonly, skiers. "I have several patients over 40 who had to stop skiing because of osteoarthritic knees," she relates. "With glucosamine sulfate, they can get back to a normal ski season." Here is her recommended regimen.

Give it time. Glucosamine sulfate may take 3 to 6 months to show results with a dosage of 500 milligrams three times a day, says Dr. Schoenbeck. The supplement is commonly available in drugstores and health food stores.

Try chondroitin. Not all osteoarthritis responds to chondroitin sulfate, another popular remedy. "The only way to know is to try," says Dr. Schoenbeck. About half of her patients with osteoarthritis say that they have less pain when they take between 250 and 500 milligrams of chondroitin sulfate three times a day in addition to their glucosamine sulfate. But, she adds, some of her patients get relief with chondroitin alone, and some report no difference.

Factor in fish. Fish-oil supplements offer the best concentration of anti-inflammatory omega-

My Mama Told Me
Does cracking your knuckles really give you arthritis?

The easy answer is, as far as we know, no. There are a couple of explanations for that sound, though. One is that cracking knuckles is actually cracking air bubbles in synovial fluid of the finger joints, like cracking air bubbles in bubble gum. Another explanation is that the sound is actually tendons snapping over a little outpouching of bone, which probably makes more sense.

There is no evidence that this practice leads to arthritis. I used to speak to groups about arthritis, and this was a common question. I'd answer by saying, "It was probably your grandmother who told you not to do it, and it was probably because it annoyed her."

While abuse and overuse of a joint can lead to arthritis, knuckle cracking is a "moment in time" pressure on the joint, not a repetitive, ongoing strain. If someone does it a couple of times a day, every day, I wouldn't be concerned. This habit is probably not going to increase anyone's risk of arthritis, given what we know today. It may just annoy those nearby.

Expert consulted
Teresa J. Brady, Ph.D.
Medical advisor
Arthritis Foundation
Atlanta

3 fatty acids, according to Dr. Schoenbeck. Her solution to swelling: 1,000 milligrams of fish oil containing EPA (eicosapentaenoic acid, a fatty acid) taken up to three times daily with food. Do not take fish oil if you have diabetes or uncontrolled high blood pressure or if you are allergic to any kind of fish. Since fish oil affects how long your body bleeds when injured, avoid if you have a bleeding disorder, take anticoagulants (blood thinners), or use aspirin regularly. Fish oil may cause nosebleeds and easy bruising as well

as upset stomach, so discontinue use if these problems occur.

Reach for relief. A former yoga teacher herself, Dr. Schoenbeck praises the art's gentle stretching as a great way to preserve flexibility and increase blood supply to the joints.

Get needled. Acupuncture, the ancient Chinese practice of inserting fine needles into the body, is winning recognition as an effective pain reliever. Two studies on osteoarthritis of the knee indicated reductions in pain and improvement in walking capabilities.

Chow down on cherries. Just 20 tart cherries a day, according to a Michigan State University study, can ease arthritis pain and inflammation. They contain substances called anthocyanins, which seem to have an antioxidant as well as an anti-inflammatory effect in joints.

Plan on pepper. The red pepper cayenne doesn't just taste hot; it brings warm relief to painful joints. Its chemicals, capsaicin and salicylates, can be rubbed on in the form of capsaicin cream. Always thoroughly wash your hands afterward to avoid getting the cream in your eyes.

Love your joints with ginger. Steep a few slivers of fresh ginger in a tea ball in one cup of freshly boiled water for 10 minutes. Let it cool to sipping temperature and drink up. It may moderate the morning aches of rheumatoid arthritis.

Soothe with green tea. Antioxidant compounds in green tea, according to research funded by the Arthritis Foundation, may ease or even prevent rheumatoid arthritis.

Defend Against Threats to the Blood Supply: Blood Health

Once upon a time, strict no-sugar diets, rigid weight-loss goals, and demanding medication regimens dominated the lives of those who had diabetes. They were told that they couldn't eat ice cream, they couldn't play sports, and they couldn't have babies. It limited their career options and their freedom. Thank goodness things have changed. Today, it's not only possible but also highly probable that people with diabetes will be able to tame their disease and live full and rewarding lives.

That's not to say that living with diabetes is easy. It complicates almost every aspect of a woman's life—career, marriage, motherhood, menopause. But with today's way of managing this disease, it is possible to achieve and enjoy a balanced, healthy lifestyle.

Unfortunately, of the approximately 8.1 million women in the United States who have some form of diabetes, up to 2.7 million of them don't know they have it and aren't receiving care.

The problem is that if diabetes isn't treated or managed properly, it can damage your vital organs, body tissues, and blood vessels, and can lead to a heart attack, stroke, or kidney, eye, and nerve damage, explains Elizabeth A. Walker, R.N., D.N.Sc. (doctor of nursing science), president of health care and education for the American Diabetes Association.

What goes wrong in your body when you have diabetes? Simply put, you have too much glucose, a type of sugar, in your blood. Your body gets glucose from the foods you eat and uses it as fuel. It is carried in the bloodstream, but it has to get into your cells before it can be expended as energy. Insulin, a hormone made by your pancreas, is the key that opens the door to let glucose into your cells, and it's usually a problem with insulin that leads to diabetes.

This disease comes in three varieties: type 1, type 2, and gestational diabetes. "In people with type 1 diabetes, the problem is decreased insulin in the pancreas, which eventually becomes *no* insulin production," says Melissa D. Katz, M.D., assistant professor of medicine in the department of endocrinology and metabolism at Weill Medical College of Cornell University in New York City. All type 1 patients must take insulin, but only some type 2 patients need to. "Type 2 diabetics produce insulin, but the amount is decreased," she says. "Type 2 patients are insulin-resistant, which means that although insulin is produced, it is not effectively taken up by the body."

Gestational diabetes involves insulin resistance as well, and it usually improves with the delivery of the baby. Diabetes can occur during pregnancy because of the mother's increased weight, which elevates insulin production, explains Dr. Katz.

Risk Factors: Type 1

Type 1, or insulin-dependent diabetes, accounts for 5 to 10 percent of all diabetes. "Both type 1 and type 2 diabetes are multifactorial," says Dr. Katz. The exact cause of type 1 diabetes is not known, but there are some identifiable risk factors.

A parent with diabetes. "The tendency to get type 1 diabetes can be inherited," says Dr. Katz. "Your risk is only slightly increased if you have a diabetic sibling."

A bug. Even if you have inherited the diabetic tendency, other environmental factors, such as illness, must come into play for it to kick in. "Certain viruses or autoimmune responses may be part of the triggering mechanism," says Dr. Katz.

Race. Type 1 diabetes is more common in Whites than in Black or Hispanic people.

Risk Factors: Type 2

If you have type 2, often called adult-onset diabetes, you're not alone. "About 95 percent of people with diabetes in this country are type 2," says Caroline Richardson, M.D., Robert Wood Johnson Clinical Scholars Fellow and lecturer in

---

THROMBOSIS

Thrombosis, or blood clotting, is a natural process that happens when you bang your arm or bump your leg, causing a blood clot or bruise to form. If it's normal, the clot will dissolve and your wound will heal. But clot formation inside healthy blood vessels is abnormal and potentially life-threatening.

The threat posed by an abnormal blood clot depends on both its size and its location. An obstructive clot in an artery of your brain, for example, can cause stroke. Blood clots in the coronary arteries to the heart are a major cause of heart attack. Blood clots in the veins to the eye can lead to loss of vision, while a clot that blocks a vein in your lungs can cause shortness of breath and even death.

Some signs of a blood clot include sudden and isolated pain in your arm or leg, followed by skin discoloration, tingling, numbness, or a cold feeling in your extremities; a hard, bluish lump in a vein; sudden or partial blindness in your eye; violent dizziness, or vertigo, that impairs your ability to stand or walk; and shortness of breath and fainting. Other blood clots often produce no obvious symptoms until it is too late.

Research shows that a tendency to have abnormal blood

---

the department of family medicine at the University of Michigan Health System in Ann Arbor. You may be at risk if one or more of the following factors apply to you.

Heritage. "There are certain populations where insulin resistance seems to be more prevalent," explains Dr. Katz. Hispanics and Blacks have about two times the rate of type 2 diabetes that Whites have, and Native Americans have a 6.3 percent higher rate than Whites.

Obesity. It seems that the genetic tendency for type 2 must be triggered by an outside force, such as excess weight. "Apple-shaped people with more upper-body fat are predisposed to insulin resistance," says Dr. Katz.

clotting can be genetic, says Alice Ma, M.D., assistant professor of hematology at the University of North Carolina in Chapel Hill.

"There are some clots that also specifically affect women, especially during pregnancy, childbirth, and the month following childbirth," she says. If a woman has a blood clot during pregnancy, she may need to be placed on blood thinners, which are safe for the baby, Dr. Ma adds.

Oral contraceptives may also increase a woman's chance of developing blood clots in her legs and may raise her risk of a pulmonary embolism, which occurs when a clot travels to the lungs. Other risk factors include smoking, a sedentary lifestyle, obesity, and surgery.

The best way to prevent abnormal blood clotting is to eat a balanced diet, get regular exercise, and drink plenty of water, particularly if you are traveling or have been immobile for a long period of time. If you're traveling by car or by plane, for example, make sure that you take time out from your trip to stretch, says Dr. Ma.

People who tend to have problems with clotting may need to be on lifelong anticoagulation that requires them to take blood thinners regularly, either intravenously or orally, Dr. Ma says.

Age. Most cases of type 2 diabetes occur in people over the age of 45, so you should start to pay particularly close attention to any warning signs at midlife.

Previous bouts of gestational diabetes. "A woman who has had gestational diabetes during one or more of her pregnancies is at an increased risk for developing type 2 diabetes later in life," says Dr. Katz. If you've had a baby who weighed 9 pounds or more at birth, your odds are further heightened.

Risk factors for gestational diabetes, which occurs in about 4 percent of all pregnancies, include obesity, a family history of maternal diabetes, and the occurrence of gestational diabetes in a previous pregnancy.

Prevention

Because the cause of type 1 diabetes is not fully understood and is thought to be both genetic and environmental, prevention may not be possible. There are large studies going on, however, that are designed to discover how to prevent both type 1 and type 2 diabetes. The best way to decrease the risk of type 2 diabetes may be with lifestyle changes, such as maintaining a normal weight, eating a lower fat diet, and getting plenty of exercise, says Dr. Walker.

Get on your feet. "A sedentary lifestyle is thought to contribute to the onset of type 2 diabetes," says Dr. Katz. Regular exercise fights insulin resistance, which makes the onset of type 2 diabetes much less likely. And if you have type 1, exercise will help keep your blood sugar levels down.

Take off some pounds. "Type 2 diabetes is much more common in obese people," says Dr. Katz. So reducing your body fat is important.

Trim the fat. A diet low in fat may help ward off diabetes. "It is thought that people with a very high fat diet are more predisposed to type 2 diabetes," Dr. Katz says.

Signs and Symptoms

If you're like a lot of women who live very full and busy lives, you're the last person you attend to; your health problems may appear at the end of your to-do list. But there are some signs and symptoms of diabetes that you should make time to watch out for. Keep in mind that type 1 symptoms usually appear suddenly, while type 2 symptoms may never show up until you develop complications.

MY MAMA TOLD ME

Can eating too much sugar give me diabetes?

Neither sugar nor carbohydrate, which is broken down into simple sugar, causes diabetes. Diabetes is really an alteration in the way we metabolize sugar—either we don't produce enough insulin, as in type 1 diabetes, or we have a resistance to the effects of insulin, as in type 2 diabetes.

Diabetes is characterized by too much glucose in the blood. Glucose is a sugar that's made by the body when carbohydrates are ingested. Diabetes exists because this metabolic process doesn't work the way it should, not because you have had too much sugar growing up.

Most experts believe that the causes of diabetes are either genetic or environmental. Overweight, physical inactivity, family history, and race/ethnicity are all risk factors for the disease.

Expert consulted
Florence Brown, M.D.
Senior staff physician
Joslin Diabetes Center
Harvard University

You're living in the bathroom. "Polyuria, or frequent or excessive urination, can be a sign of type 1 or 2 diabetes," says Dr. Katz. Polyuria is dangerous because it can worsen the already present dehydration from the disease, she says.

You're chugging water. Polydipsia, or excessive thirst, is another sign of type 1 or 2 diabetes. The thirst is related to the fluid lost because of polyuria.

Your world is fuzzy. Blurry vision can indicate the presence of type 1 or 2 diabetes. "High levels of circulating blood glucose can cause a distortion of the lens," explains Dr. Katz.

You're getting frequent and stubborn infections. Type 2 diabetes can cause repeated or hard-to-cure infections in the body on account of the increased levels of sugar in the blood. Infections typically attack the skin, gums, vagina, or bladder.

You're losing lots of weight. Type 1 diabetes often causes sudden and extreme weight loss.

Don't Panic!

Taken collectively, the symptoms of diabetes are pretty classic, says Florence Brown, M.D., senior staff physician at the Joslin Diabetes Center at Harvard University. "If anything, the problem with diabetes tends to be that the diagnosis is sometimes missed." The symptoms taken separately could point to other ailments, says Dr. Brown. Sudden, unexplained weight loss could point to an overactive thyroid gland. Blurry vision, particularly in those over 40, could be a sign of aging-related changes. And excessive urination could point to a urinary tract infection. If you have only one or two symptoms, you should probably still be checked for diabetes, particularly if you have some of the risk factors.

But even if you discover that you have diabetes, there is no need to panic, says Dr. Brown. It's not that horrible of a diagnosis—after all, there are things that you can do about it.

Who Do I See?

If you've been diagnosed with type 1 or 2 diabetes, there are a number of experts whom you can see for care. You may choose to visit your primary-care physician first. "Most people with diabetes never see a diabetes specialist, who is usually an endocrinologist," says Dr. Richardson. Primary-care doctors are usually well-trained at managing type 2 diabetes, and many also treat type 1 patients.

"Some cases of diabetes are more difficult to manage than others," says Dr. Richardson. "If the patient and primary-care doctor both feel that the diabetes management is not working as well as it should, a consultation with an endocrinologist may help."

Nurse educators and nutritionists specializing in diabetes management can address all of the different behaviors involved in managing diabetes, says Dr. Richardson. A nurse educator will help you learn how to check your blood sugar levels, take your medication properly, and monitor your diet.

Whether you have type 1 or type 2 diabetes, you may be prone to secondary symptoms requiring a visit to other specialty physicians. If you have coronary artery disease, you should see a cardiologist, says Dr. Katz. You may also need to see a nephrologist for kidney problems. "I recommend that all diabetes patients see an ophthalmologist twice a year so any possible retinal disease is caught early," she says. Periodic visits to a podiatrist are also helpful because decreased sensation in the feet can lead to unrecognized cuts and infections.

"For patients with type 2 diabetes who do not exercise or walk regularly, the most important

WOMEN ASK WHY

Why did my mom have to take insulin injections for her diabetes, while the doctor tells me I only need to diet and exercise to control mine?

Today, we know more about the benefits of dietary management and exercise in managing diabetes than we did 20 years ago. We know that people can lose just 10 to 15 pounds and improve their glucose control, whereas years ago, doctors would just automatically use insulin to manage the disease.

The sad thing is that many people think of diabetes as an all-or-nothing proposition. They've been told or they mistakenly believe that they have to lose a great deal of weight and curb their diets to the point of deprivation in order to attain a healthy outcome. Many health professionals talk in terms of 100 percent compliance, meaning that the patient must do everything correctly 100 percent of the time. But that may not be necessary to improve your blood sugar.

According to the American Heart Association and the American Diabetes Association, if people can lose 10 percent of their weight, or an average of 15 pounds, they will improve blood pressure, cholesterol, and blood sugar. The bottom line is, don't be overwhelmed. Focus on small goals. And even if you have to use medication, you may even be able to come off it once you lose some weight and begin exercising and eating a healthy diet.

It's important for people to diet and exercise so that they can better utilize the insulin that their bodies make and perhaps put off the need for extra insulin in the future.

Expert consulted
Gail D'Eramo Melkus, Ed.D.
Associate professor and nurse practitioner
Yale School of Nursing

consultant might be a personal trainer," says Dr. Richardson. "Personal trainers are experts in helping sedentary patients become physically active." If you cannot afford a personal trainer, you can join an exercise class or exercise with a group of friends for added motivation.

What Can I Expect?

When I first was diagnosed with diabetes, I thought I was dying, recalls former Miss America Nicole Johnson, who has type 1 diabetes. "But once I better educated myself about the disease, I learned that I could control it," she says. Although a diagnosis of type 1 or 2 diabetes will necessitate some lifestyle changes, it is possible to live a happy, healthy life with the disease.

Whether you have type 1 or 2 diabetes, you will need to keep your blood sugar level as close to normal as possible. If you have type 1, and possibly if you have type 2, you will need to take insulin, probably by self-injection. Your physician or nurse will tell you how much insulin you need, when to take it, and what kind you should take. "Instead of injecting insulin, you may also be put on an insulin pump," says Dr. Katz. The size of a beeper, the pump delivers insulin into your abdomen through a small catheter. "The pump gives you a basal level of insulin at all times, but you can program it to give more in preparation for a meal or exercise," she says.

Controlling your blood sugar will require following a meal plan that will tell you when and how much to eat. "Nutrition is very important in the management of both type 1 and type 2 diabetes," says Dr. Katz. The regimen will likely be somewhat more strict if you have type 1.

A diagnosis of type 1 diabetes will also require

WOMAN TO WOMAN
Determination Is Key

Nicole Johnson has lived with diabetes for more than 7 years. As Miss America 1999, Johnson, 26, travels tens of thousands of miles a year, encouraging people to learn more about the disease. Her message to people with diabetes is a simple one: Stay in control and don't give up.

When I first learned that I had diabetes, I was devastated. I thought I was dying.

At the time, I was in college, working a part-time job, juggling extracurricular activities and volunteer work. On weekends, I was starting to compete in the Miss America program, hoping to win scholarships to help pay for school.

When the doctors finally realized that I had type 1 diabetes, I had to drop out of school and stop all my other activities. I learned that to survive, I had to rely on a constant stream of insulin and test my blood glucose regularly.

I was told that I couldn't drink soda and would never be able to eat desserts again. I was afraid I might never be able to marry or have children. I thought a high-pressure career like journalism would be difficult at best. And winning a major beauty pageant? I wasn't the only one who had

you to monitor your blood sugar level. You will do this by pricking your finger and testing your blood with a kit that will indicate your sugar level. You may also need to do home tests if you have a more severe case of type 2 diabetes.

An exercise routine will likely be prescribed for you whether you have type 1 or type 2 diabetes. Exercise helps your body use blood sugar and, therefore, lowers glucose levels in your blood. If you have type 2, exercise will probably be prescribed in conjunction with a weight-loss plan to keep blood sugar levels in check.

On top of everything else, diabetes can

doubts. Many people told me my goals and dreams were impossible.

For months, I felt fear, self-pity, and anger. Why me? How did I get this? What will happen to me next? There were a million different questions, and as I learned more about diabetes, there seemed to be almost as many answers.

Soon, I made up my mind that even though I might not be able to beat the disease, I wasn't going to let it beat me.

So I read everything I could about diabetes. I found support groups. I learned about the role of diet, nutrition, and exercise in helping to manage my illness. And not only was I able to go back to school, I doubled up on my classes and went on to graduate school.

I worked a part-time job, landed an internship in broadcasting, and returned to pageant competition.

It took me five tries to win the state title that would get me to the Miss America pageant. Some told me that I would never win because of my diabetes. But in 1999, I was crowned Miss America.

I tell people with diabetes that the most important thing that they can do is to be tested and educated. Then, when you have information, you have to take it upon yourself to become an active part of your medical team and to be proactive in your own care.

Don't deny your illness. Most people go through a denial stage when they are first diagnosed, but a long-term state of denial can be dangerous. If you find yourself saying things like "One bite won't hurt," or if you stop doing necessary procedures such as testing your blood sugar, you may be in a state of denial. To help yourself get back on track, write down your care plan and goals along with reasons why they are important.

Relieve some stress. The stress of diabetes management can be overwhelming, but there are ways to reduce it. Sharing with members of a support group can help. Sometimes, adding positive things to your life, such as starting an exercise program, taking dance lessons, or volunteering at a charity, can also help.

Don't give up. When you have unexpected highs and lows, keep in mind that your blood sugar level is controlled by outside factors as well as your own efforts. Medications, illnesses, and major life events can all interfere.

worsen changes associated with menopause, such as a lack of sexual desire, vaginal dryness, and pain during intercourse. If you're menstruating or menopausal, you may find that your blood sugar is going haywire.

Coping with diabetes, as with any chronic illness, can be challenging both physically and emotionally. Managing diabetes is a full-time job that calls on your ability to constantly motivate yourself to do the things that will keep you healthy. There are some things that experts suggest you can do to help keep your mind and body in shape.

Conventional Wisdom

Diabetes is treated with food plans, exercise, oral medications known as insulin sensitizers, or insulin injections. The goal of treatment is to keep blood glucose levels as close to normal as possible.

Besides relying on diet and exercise, people with diabetes have to make time to monitor their blood sugar levels. With diabetes, the doctor and patient set a target blood glucose range, which may be slightly different from the normal range. Performing regular tests helps ensure that you

IRON-DEFICIENCY ANEMIA

You've probably seen the commercials on television: a young woman or mother complaining that she's fatigued, run-down, or can't get enough sleep—the announcer saying that an iron supplement is the answer to her prayers.

But in reality, iron-deficiency anemia is overdiagnosed, says Suzanne Swietnicki, M.D., of the Mayo Clinic in Jacksonville, Florida. "Iron is overprescribed, in general, in the United States. Largely because of a lot of vitamin ads, people seem to think that when they are tired, they need to take iron. But taking iron can be unhealthy unless you have a reason beyond just feeling tired."

Iron-deficiency anemia, the most common type of anemia, is the lack of iron in the blood. The most common reason for iron deficiency is heavy menstruation, usually lasting longer than 7 days. It can also be caused by blood loss, poor diet, an increased need for iron, or an underlying medical condition. Pregnancy also increases the risk of iron-deficiency anemia. Iron deficiency doesn't always lead to anemia, but it can cause other problems, such as fatigue and weakened immunity.

In most cases, women are not aware that they are anemic. In severe cases, however, you may feel extreme fatigue and weakness, dizziness or fainting, shortness of breath, or heart palpitations. Other symptoms include pale skin, pale nailbeds, and pale lower eyelids.

In addition, several groups of women including those of Mediterranean, Indian, and African-American descent may have a genetic anemia, called thalassemia, which can be misdiagnosed as iron-deficiency anemia.

Health-care professionals don't usually recommend iron supplements unless iron deficiency is confirmed. In fact, excess iron can be harmful because it can lead to liver and heart disease. If you have been diagnosed specifically with iron-deficiency anemia, however, an iron supplement may be prescribed.

The best prevention is to eat a balanced diet containing iron-rich foods, such as meat; fish; poultry; green vegetables, like broccoli and spinach; and legumes, like beans and peas.

meet your blood glucose goals. "Monitoring your blood sugar and having that information is a powerful tool. It allows you to control your diabetes and not let your diabetes control you," says Dr. Brown.

It is also important for people with diabetes to control the levels of fats in their blood. High cholesterol and triglyceride levels can lead to other serious health problems, such as heart disease and stroke. Blood fats are controlled by some of the same things that control blood glucose levels: healthy eating and exercise.

If following a food-and-exercise plan isn't enough for you to reach and maintain blood glucose goals, the next step in diabetes treatment is to add blood glucose–lowering medications that come in pill form. These oral medications, called insulin sensitizers, are used in conjunction with a healthy diet and exercise to enhance treatment.

Great Alternatives

With the number of people who have diabetes surging, health food stores and experts in holistic medicine are offering a greater variety of supplements to aid glucose management. The following are some of the more common alternative treatments recommended by Jill Stanard, N.D., a naturopathic physician practicing in Providence, Rhode Island.

Gymnema. The leaves of this plant, which grows in tropical forests of central and southern India, seem to help control blood glucose levels. A dose of 400 milligrams a day is recommended.

Bilberry and ginkgo. Both bilberry and ginkgo may improve circulation, lowering the risk of eye damage in patients with diabetes. They are both available freeze-dried or as a tincture. Follow the manufacturer's directions. Do not use ginkgo with antidepressant MAO inhibitor drugs such as phenelzine sulfate (Nardil) or tranylcypromine (Parnate), aspirin or other nonsteroidal anti-inflammatory medications, or blood-thinning medications such as warfarin (Coumadin). Ginkgo can cause dermatitis, diarrhea, and vomiting in doses higher than 240 milligrams of concentrated extract.

Vitamins. "Vitamin C can help prevent the damage to blood vessels that accompanies diabetes," says Dr. Stanard. Take 500 milligrams in the morning and another 500 milligrams later in the day. Take 400 IU of vitamin E daily to help prevent blood vessel damage and help cells use insulin. Niacin contributes to improved insulin activity, and 100 micrograms per day when combined with 200 micrograms of chromium may help normalize glucose levels. Doses above 35 milligrams must be taken under medical supervision.

As with any kind of treatment, you should consult with your doctor or other health professional before using any herbal or alternative treatment.

Support Your Infrastructure: Bone Health

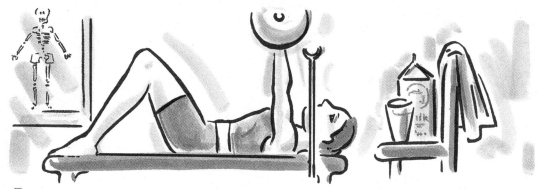

argaret Atwood, the Canadian novelist, poet, and critic, once said, "The basic Female body comes with the following accessories: garter belt, panti-girdle, crinoline, camisole, bustle, brassiere, stomacher, chemise, virgin zone, spike heels, nose ring, veil, kid gloves, fishnet stockings, fichu, bandeau, Merry Widow, weepers, chokers, barrettes, bangles, beads, lorgnette, feather boa, basic black, compact, Lycra stretch one-piece with modesty panel, designer peignoir, flannel nightie, lace teddy, bed, head."

An exhaustive list, but she may have missed one item: a plaster cast for those with a tendency toward brittle bones.

The disease of "porous bone," osteoporosis, can strike at any age but prefers postmenopausal women. That's because estrogen, which has a starring role in maintaining bone strength, begins to dwindle around menopause, making you more susceptible. Osteoporosis is a stealthy disease and has no symptoms of its own. In fact, the first clue that your bones are fragile may not come until you break one, usually in the wrist, hip, or spine, during a bump or fall. In time, it

can make your bones so brittle that you find yourself hunched over with a dowager's hump.

All in all, not a pretty picture, but not an inevitable one either. In fact, the outlook for this disease is improving all the time.

"The media picture of the older woman is of one bent over and disabled," notes Karen A. Roberto, Ph.D., professor and director of the Center for Gerontology at Virginia Polytechnic Institute and State University in Blacksburg, Virginia. While osteoporosis can disfigure and disable, that's absolutely not the picture of everyone with the disease, she says. "We have new treatment options, and there's new hope."

The hope is that osteoporosis, which sneaks around our skeletons like a cat burglar, can be caught before it makes off with the strength and support of our bones.

Risk Factors

Although there's nothing we can do about some of the major risk factors for osteoporosis, others are well within our control. So while it may be impossible to make this disease disappear from the face of the Earth, each of us can make some changes to help keep it from becoming a scourge in her life.

Here are the risk factors we're just plain stuck with, according to the Osteoporosis and Related Bone Diseases unit of the National Institutes of Health.

Gender. Eight out of 10 Americans with low bone density or osteoporosis are women. In their lifetimes, fully half of all women over age 50 will have broken bones as a result of the disease.

Age. It's true that risk increases as the years roll on: time steals bone strength and density. The lowered estrogen levels of menopause, combined with age, are "the biggest influences on what happens to a woman's bones," according to Ethel S. Siris, M.D., director of the Toni Stabile Center for the Prevention and Treatment of Osteoporosis at Columbia-Presbyterian Medical Center in New York City.

Body size. If you're small-boned and thin (under 127 pounds), you're at greater risk than bigger women.

Race. Caucasian and Asian women have been thought to be at higher risk than African-American and Hispanic women. A study from Columbia University, though, suggests that ethnic background is a less important factor than many believed.

Family and personal history. You're more susceptible to breaking a bone if one of your parents has a

---

BAD TO THE BONE: STEROIDS

Remember the schoolyard retort "Sticks and stones may break my bones, but names will never hurt me"? There's one name that may: steroid-user.

Corticosteroid drugs like prednisone (Deltasone) or dexamethasone (Decadron) are often prescribed for people with rheumatoid arthritis, asthma, lung disease, and other chronic ailments. But even as they help with the symptoms of those diseases, they can be paving the way for osteoporosis.

"We have to be especially watchful with people who are taking steroids, because we know that the medication can cause bone loss," says Diana L. Anderson, Ph.D., director of the osteoporosis center at St. Paul Medical Center in Dallas. Some 20 percent of the people who come to her center, she reports, are taking some form of steroids, increasing their risk of fractures.

And the risk can be big. According to the National Osteoporosis Foundation, taking corticosteroids is among the top 10 risk factors for developing the bone-sapping disease. The bone loss from steroids can be swift, especially in the first 3 to 6 months of treatment. "If you take steroids, you need to be aware of the effect on your bones," says Dr. Anderson. Most of the men treated at the St. Paul Osteoporosis Center are referred by their rheumatologists because of steroid usage, she reports. Both women and men who have had heart or lung transplants are often referred, according to the director, because some of their medications can also rob bone.

Bones fall prey to steroids for two reasons: first, the drugs chip away at the body's bone-making power, and second, they impede the absorption of calcium, a vital bone-building nutrient.

Here is Dr. Anderson's bone-healthy advice for women who take steroids.

Know your steroid status. Talk with your doctor about your medications and the effect that they may have on your skeleton.

Remember the two Ms. Your higher risk means that you should be managed and monitored carefully.

history of fractures or if you've had a fracture as an adult.

Here are the risk factors that you can do something about.

Sex hormones. Due to low estrogen levels, an abnormal absence of menstrual periods, including a premenopausal halt in menstruation due to anorexia, bulimia, or too much exercise, can boost risk. So can normal or early menopause.

Bone-depleting diet. Have you made a lifelong habit of skimping on calcium and vitamin D? You could be in trouble.

Medications. Drugs used to treat chronic medical conditions such as rheumatoid arthritis and seizures can batter bones. Other risk boosters include thyroid hormones, glucocorticoids, anticonvulsants, and antacids with aluminum.

Smoking. If you still need a reason to quit, think about this: By smoking, you double your risk of an osteoporosis bone break. The habit has been linked to earlier menopause, bone cell damage, and blockage of new bone.

Excessive drinking. Heavy alcohol use is not a healthy habit, especially in the eyes of the National Osteoporosis Foundation (NOF). Drinking too much will increase your risk of developing the disease.

Inertia. "If you're physically active, you avoid the extra bone loss that highly sedentary people get," advises Dr. Siris. So get moving.

High blood pressure. In a study of 3,676 women ages 66 to 91, doctors found that the higher the blood pressure, the greater the amount of bone loss in the hip, which means an increased risk of fracture there.

REAL-LIFE SCENARIO

She Won't Get Her Bone Density Checked Because She's Scared of What She'll Find Out

Jo, 55, knows all about osteoporosis. She's made it her business to know. Both her mother and her grandmother suffered terrible leg and rib fractures from the disease after they went through menopause, and she has no intention of ending up the same way. So she has read every bit of literature she could find on the subject, has been adding extra calcium to her diet for years, and does weight-bearing, bone-building exercise religiously. But now that she's gone through menopause herself, her doctor has recommended that she get her bone density checked, and she has adamantly refused. As far as she's concerned, she has done everything as "natural" as she can to protect herself, and if she's going to end up like her mother and grandmother anyway, she doesn't want to know until it happens. Should her doctor just give up?

In Jo's case, it's what she might *not* find out that's disturbing. Without a bone-density test, Jo and her doctor can't know exactly what her bone mass picture is now, and they'll have nothing to compare it with in the future.

Far from giving up, her doctor should tell Jo why this test is so important: It gives a baseline reading. It gives knowledge. And the doctor can use that knowledge to Jo's advantage in future tests to detect bone loss, can prescribe medications, and can recommend changes in exercise or diet—all to help slow down or even halt osteoporosis.

Prevention

You *can* beat the odds of getting osteoporosis, say experts. These are the leading strategies, according to Felicia Cosman, M.D., clinical director of the NOF.

Reduce your risk. If you have one or more of the risk factors that can be changed, change it. If you smoke, stop. Cut down on heavy

So while Jo is smart to take extra calcium and do weight-bearing exercise, she's hurting herself by avoiding the test. Her doctor may be able to win her over by explaining how simple, fast, and noninvasive a bone-density test is.

The preferred bone-density test, and the one that's most precise, is a DEXA (dual-energy x-ray absorptiometry). There's nothing scary, no enclosure, no pain; the test is totally nonthreatening, and you often can keep all your clothes on.

Here's what happens: You lie on a regular doctor's exam table in your street clothes (as long as you're wearing no metal, like a buckle or bra fastener). An arm called a scanner is positioned above you, and it moves back and forth over you, from your neck to your lower abdomen. While this happens, a technician is usually in the room with you, watching the images that the scanner feeds to a computer screen. This equipment is very sensitive and high-tech.

After 15 minutes on the table, you're done. A DEXA test is quite safe: the scanner emits less radiation than one chest x-ray. There's no lead-lined room or special radiation requirement because the DEXA test is so low-dose.

To a great degree, osteoporosis is preventable. What Jo doesn't know can hurt her, and her doctor should try even harder to convince her to get a DEXA test.

Expert consulted
Diane L. Anderson, Ph.D.
Director of the osteoporosis center
St. Paul Medical Center
Dallas

drinking. If you're taking any medications that may damage bone, talk to your doctor about possibly reducing dosage or changing medications (but don't make any changes without consulting your doctor first). If you have low estrogen, consider hormone-replacement therapy (HRT). Get your blood pressure under control. And of course, if you don't exercise, get moving.

Concentrate on calcium. Bone-building calcium comes from an array of dairy foods (nonfat or low-fat), calcium-fortified soy milk and juices, and supplements. Don't rely on pills alone, though, to get your 1,200 to 1,500 milligrams daily. "It's important that your diet plus any supplement provide at least 1,200 milligrams of calcium every day," advises Dr. Cosman.

But not just any calcium supplement will do. Read the label to find the elemental calcium content, says Dr. Cosman. That's the important number to know if you want to meet your daily need. A 1,000-milligram calcium carbonate pill, for example, may have just 400 milligrams of elemental calcium content. For best absorption, look for calcium citrate.

Dig into "D." Because vitamin D helps the body absorb calcium, it's a grade-A part of avoiding osteoporosis. Get 400 IU per day in a multivitamin, a vitamin D supplement, or a calcium supplement. Dr. Cosman suggests taking even more vitamin D if you're over 65 (but keep it below 2,000 IU). Vitamin D and calcium are a powerful pair: They've been shown to significantly reduce the risk of hip and other fractures in women over age 65.

Stand up for your bones. Aerobic exercise done while standing appears to yield the most bone benefits, according to Dr. Cosman. Tennis, a treadmill workout, walking, stair-climbing, and low-impact aerobic dance are all recommended. Add in a muscle-strengthening routine with free weights or an exercise video and repeat three to five times per week. You'll help keep bones and muscles strong, boost co-

WOMEN ASK WHY

Why should I care about what illnesses my father had? Aren't I supposed to take after my mother?

It's true that if you have a parent with osteoporosis—and it's generally your mother—you're at increased risk for getting the disease as well. But you can't just look at your mother and say, "Well, she was okay, so I will be, too."

It's important to know whether your father has osteoporosis because family history is a prime risk factor. Men are less likely to get osteoporosis than women. They represent 20 percent of those affected, but they are by no means immune. Unlike women, men don't have a sudden change in estrogen that leads to rapid loss of bone mass. They lose bone mass over years and years, especially if they don't have adequate calcium intake and they're over the age of 35.

We're really not sure exactly how much a father's genetic legacy influences his children's susceptibility to the disease, but we do know that if either of your parents has osteoporosis, you are at risk. So even though osteoporosis occurs much more often in women than men, the genetic risk factors make it wise to know the status of *both* parents.

Expert consulted
Sicy H. Lee, M.D.
Assistant clinical professor of medicine
New York University School of Medicine
New York City

ordination, and probably reduce your risk of falling, she says.

Drink to your health? Moderate amounts of alcohol—say, one glass of wine a day—may actually be good for your bones (except for women at high risk of breast cancer), reports Dr. Cosman. In a study of 188 postmenopausal women, researchers found that those who drank at least the equivalent of about one glass of wine daily had higher bone densities than those who abstained. Exactly how alcohol helps is still a question mark; it may increase estrogen or stimulate the body's production of calcitonin, a bone-friendly hormone.

Get tested. For women at or beyond menopause who have one or more risk factors or who have had a fracture, the cornerstone of prevention is three letters: BMD. They stand for bone mineral density, also called bone mass, and having it measured is a must, especially if you have a family history of osteoporosis. Dr. Siris recommends that you have your BMD tested when you turn 65 or if you're postmenopausal, whichever comes first.

"Just as a mammogram gives you a baseline for detecting breast cancer, a BMD test is your foundation for detecting and preventing osteoporosis," says Diane L. Anderson, Ph.D., director of the osteoporosis center at St. Paul Medical Center in Dallas. The object is to detect the disease before a fracture occurs, predict your chances of a future break, and monitor rates of bone loss. Several types of machines are used to measure bone density, but the undisputed leader is DEXA (dual-energy x-ray absorptiometry).

"DEXA is the gold standard of bone-density testing," says Dr. Anderson, who describes the process as painless, noninvasive, and brief: 15 minutes. With very low dose radiation, it scans your spine and hip to take "pictures" of these areas where osteoporosis can have the gravest consequences.

Other devices take bone-mass measurements

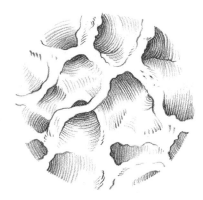

In healthy bone, the network of numerous bone fragments is large and connected, giving strength and stability.

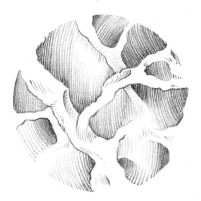

This bone, riddled with osteoporosis, shows bone fragments that are sparse and not well-connected.

in your wrist, heel, or finger, and an ultrasound version takes readings at your heel, shinbone, and kneecap.

A handful of medications are available for preventing osteoporosis, some fairly new, but they are for postmenopausal women only, according to Dr. Siris.

Signs and Symptoms

Are you peering a little higher over the steering wheel lately? Do you have a backache that doesn't go away? Or have you had a broken bone after age 40? These are all warning signs that osteoporosis could be doing its bone-zapping work.

Shrinking stature. Up to an inch of height loss is common among those ages 60 to 80, but if you are younger or have shrunk more than that, it could be due to a spinal fracture caused by osteoporosis. Such fractures can be gradual or can strike suddenly. "You may have sudden, severe pain with a vertebral fracture that gets better over several weeks," observes Dr. Siris. More common is a gradual break in a vertebra—"it kind of squishes down on itself," she says—and either one can make you shorter.

An aching back. Chronic, nagging back pain can be a warning sign of a fractured vertebra. "The break changes the contour of the back, and you're not aligned properly," notes Dr. Siris.

A fracture from a fall. If you slip on the stairs and break your wrist, the fracture might not be due to osteoporosis, but it could be. The NOF estimates that osteoporosis causes more than 1.5 million fractures every year. Weakened bones are simply more susceptible to breaking than strong ones. And if you've had an osteoporotic fracture after age 40, you're twice as likely to have another as someone who hasn't had one at all.

"Many middle-aged and older people think, 'Well, I get older and I fall,'" says Dr. Anderson. "But it isn't the falling down that really causes the fractures. It's the osteoporosis."

Naturally, preventing falls is a prime objective if you have osteoporosis. Here are some everyday tips that can help.

Slip into shoe safety. Stick with supportive, low-heeled shoes, indoors and out; rubber soles increase traction. Avoid walking in socks, stockings, or slippers.

Walk wisely. When sidewalks are slippery, keep on the grass. Step carefully on highly polished floors, especially when they're wet.

Clean up your rooms. Clear the clutter, especially on floors, that invites bumps and stumbles.

Keep floor fashions secure. Use area rugs and carpets with nonskid backs.

Head off bathroom hazards. Put safety first with a rubber bath mat in the tub or shower, and install grab bars nearby.

Cut the cord. Let a cordless phone cut out those headlong rushes to answer calls.

Don't Panic!

These pains and problems may trigger false fears of osteoporosis, according to Dr. Siris.

Intermittent back pain. The most likely cause is a muscle sprain or possibly arthritis. Osteoporosis itself doesn't hurt, so there's no painful alarm to warn of thinning bones. "If a bone breaks suddenly because of osteoporosis, then of course there's pain," observes Dr. Siris. But the disease doesn't declare itself until that break.

Curving upper back. "Some women come to me because they think they're starting to get a curved back, the dreaded dowager's hump, and they're terrified," Dr. Siris says. What many actually have is a slight bend to the upper back from poor posture or a muscle condition unrelated to osteoporosis.

Who Do I See?

Since osteoporosis is a "woman's disease," the first health professional to bring up the topic may be a gynecologist. "Gynecologists are becoming more responsible and responsive about

---

PAGET'S DISEASE: LEGACY OF THE MAYFLOWER

Along with its cargo of pilgrims and dreams, the Mayflower may also have brought to America a genetic legacy that deforms bones. It's called Paget's disease, named after the English physician who first studied it, Sir James Paget.

Like osteoporosis, Paget's disease involves bone cells called osteoclasts that remove old bone so that other cells can build new bone. Unlike osteoporosis, which can affect the entire skeleton, Paget's osteoclasts zero in on the skull, spine, pelvis, or legs, creating enlarged bones that are weaker than normal. Pain, deformities, fractures, and arthritis can follow.

"In Paget's, the osteoclasts at affected sites aggressively remove bone," relates Ethel S. Siris, M.D., director of the Toni Stabile Center for the Prevention and Treatment of Osteoporosis at Columbia-Presbyterian Medical Center in New York City. "That requires the bone-building cells to come marching in in great numbers and quickly, haphazardly, lay down new bone." The resulting new bone is bigger but flimsier than usual. And the outcome in more severe cases can be an enlarged skull, sometimes with hearing loss from affected nerves; a bowed leg; or a curved spine. What's the

---

educating their patients, as are some internists," says Dr. Cosman.

As the NOF works to spread awareness, women themselves are taking the lead. "We're telling women that if you're menopausal—and especially if you have any of the risk factors—you should talk to your primary-care physician about getting a bone-density test," says Dr. Cosman. Often, it's this patient-to-doctor inquiry, and not vice versa, that leads to testing.

Osteoporosis doesn't "belong" to any one medical specialty, so if an expert is needed, there are three main types who may be called on. One, like Dr. Cosman, is an endocrinologist, who

Mayflower connection? Paget's is very common in England, present in other parts of Europe, and rare in Asia and Africa.

Affecting about 2 percent of Americans over the age of 50, Paget's can run in families, says Dr. Siris, and research is pinpointing genes that may be responsible. Viruses are also suspected in the ailment. Women and men are equally affected by the disease, which can be very mild. Many people with the disorder don't know they have it.

Osteoclasts aren't the only thing that Paget's disease and osteoporosis have in common. "A lot of the drugs that some people think are new for osteoporosis were actually being used years ago for Paget's," says Dr. Siris. Calcitonin and bisphosphonates such as alendronate (Fosamax) or risedronate (Actonel), which work on shutting down overzealous bone removal, were the drugs of choice as long as 25 years ago.

Today, blood tests, x-rays, and bone scans tell physicians whether Paget's is at work and where. "This disease doesn't strike an array of places in the skeleton like osteoporosis," says Dr. Siris. "Where it's detected is where it is." While research moves forward to identify just what causes Paget's, drugs and exercise therapies can help allay pain and the progress of the disease. "A lot of primary-care physicians still say, 'Forget it, there's no treatment,'" she says. "That's just not true."

deals with hormone-related conditions. Another is a rheumatologist, who concentrates on diseases of joints and connective tissue. Finally, orthopedists are doctors who correct skeletal problems surgically.

What Can I Expect?

If you can avoid fractures, you'll evade the pain potential of osteoporosis. "If you've never broken a bone," says Dr. Siris, "you can expect that with proper evaluation and intervention you'll be able to maintain good bone health as you grow older."

But if you're in that half of women over age 50 who have an osteoporotic break in their lifetimes, the picture changes. You may recover to as good as new from a first spinal fracture, according to Dr. Siris, but your risk of future fractures zooms. A hip break requires surgery, whereas a broken arm or wrist can be put in a cast.

Emotional fractures can't be detected by a machine, but they can be as shattering as a broken bone, says Dr. Roberto. "Osteoporosis affects every aspect of a woman's life, from physical pain and disability rolling right into self-esteem and self-perception."

After 15 years researching the psychological and social aspects of the disease, Dr. Roberto finds that women's feelings about osteoporosis move through three stages: denial, information-seeking, and coping.

Denial, or a dismissive attitude, often comes with the second fracture: "The first fracture, most women manage; the second fracture can begin a spiral into fear, depression, and stress," she says.

In the information-seeking stage, the woman herself gathers all the material she can about osteoporosis. Dr. Roberto says that family and friends need to be included in this information loop, too. "We've found that when a woman has a visible fracture, like a broken hip, the family is usually helpful and understanding. But when it's a vertebral fracture, which you can't see," she relates, "the attitude can be 'Mom looks the same; what's the problem?'"

Finally, coping comes as a woman readapts to the reality that there are things she can do and things she can't, says Dr. Roberto. One woman who loved marathon shopping days parcelled her outings to one store per day, with rest days in between. Others, who had been skiers or golfers, took up less vigorous activities. "Our runners became our walkers," she says.

Based on interviews with hundreds of women with osteoporosis, Dr. Roberto offers these coping strategies.

Find strength in numbers. Support groups can be a great source of comfort and assurance. If your doctor can't help you locate one nearby, write to the National Osteoporosis Foundation, Attn.: Support Groups, 1232 22nd Street NW, Washington, DC 20037-1292 or visit the foundation's Web site.

Cultivate calm and quiet. Relaxation techniques like meditation and visualization can help ease fear and stress.

Opt for options. When pain alters your plans, find a distraction: read, talk to a friend on the phone, work on a craft project.

Be frank with family. Some older women with osteoporosis have a particular emotional stab: They can't pick up their grandchildren for fear of breaking a bone. Letting children and adults in the family know what you're experiencing helps them understand.

Conventional Wisdom

Advances in detecting and treating the disease help make it far from inevitable. Here are some of those strategies.

Determining density. In the last few years, techniques to measure bone density have multiplied, says Dr. Cosman. While the DEXA test of the hip and spine is considered the best, other

WOMEN ASK WHY

Why is a fractured hip so serious for an older woman?

A fractured or broken hip means surgery, and to some extent, that's why it's so serious: the complications of surgery and of being immobilized.

At the National Osteoporosis Foundation, we have a single statistic that points out just how grave this can be: an average of 24 percent of hip fracture patients age 50 and over die in the year following their fractures. Just as alarming, about 25 percent of older women with hip fractures require placement in a nursing home because they never regain the independence that they had prior to the fractures. When you consider that women have a hip fracture rate two to three times higher than men and that 80 percent of Americans with osteoporosis are women, it's clear that this poses a considerable threat to our gender.

Older people should stay active to maintain health, but a hip fracture can keep them bedridden for a week or two. Subject them to surgery, and there's a great toll from that: They can get pneumonia, heart disease, or infections, and all of this contributes to the death rate in the year after the fracture. The majority survive, but quality of life can be severely af-

tests can still be useful in predicting the risk of fracture.

Some "peripheral" tests, like those found at health fairs, can be helpful screening tools, notes Dr. Anderson. "They may tell you if you have osteoporosis or a bone density that should be looked at with a DEXA, but not all of these tests are equal in their ability to predict the risk of fractures."

Hormone power. For postmenopausal women, hormone-replacement therapy with estrogen or other hormones is still a standby in reducing the risk of osteoporotic fractures. But questions about side effects and links with cancer remain unresolved.

fected. Hip fracture is a leading cause of admission to nursing homes.

Actually, when we say "hip fracture," we're really talking about a break in the thighbone, or femur. The top of the femur, called the proximal femur, is where "hip fracture" occurs—it's all the same bone. That bone is what fits into the socket of the hip, like an upside-down L—the short piece is actually in the hip and the long piece is the thighbone. So what most people call a broken hip, doctors call a proximal femur fracture. And a fracture along any part of the femur is a major problem; it always requires surgery.

From my clinical experience, I can report a common scenario: Women in their seventies and eighties who are fully functional and having a good quality of life fall and fracture their hips. Many of them just never get back to life as before because the older you get, the harder it is to recover from a trauma. Put a 20-year-old down for 2 weeks, and she pops back up, but this is less and less likely as people get older.

Sadly, statistically, a hip fracture is what's going to take many older women down.

Expert consulted
Felicia Cosman, M.D.
Clinical director
National Osteoporosis Foundation

Pharmacy factor. New drugs with fewer side effects are now available to prevent and treat osteoporosis. They include raloxifene (Evista), a selective estrogen receptor modulator (SERM) shown to increase bone mass in the spine and hips and reduce the risk of vertebral fracture by up to 50 percent. A 3-year study of 7,705 postmenopausal women that produced those results also suggested a stunning effect on breast cancer: raloxifene reduced the risk of invasive breast cancer by 75 percent.

Also making a difference are alendronate (Fosamax), which is especially effective for reducing spine and hip fractures, and a companion drug called risedronate (Actonel). Calcitonin, a hormone that slows bone loss and modestly builds spinal bone density, is a common treatment for women at least 5 years beyond menopause.

Great Alternatives

Calcium and vitamin D: there's no contest and no controversy here between conventional and alternative medicine. These are the big guns in the battle to keep bones strong, agrees Lorilee Schoenbeck, N.D., a naturopathic physician in Shelburne, Vermont.

Once a patient's bone-density test indicates osteopenia (reduced bone mass that isn't yet osteoporosis), Dr. Schoenbeck tailors these options to her individual needs.

Boost calcium benefits. To ensure that the calcium you take is readily absorbed into your system, Dr. Schoenbeck suggests that you look for calcium citrate supplements. Shoot for 1,000 milligrams as your total daily intake of calcium if you're premenopausal and 1,500 milligrams a day if you're postmenopausal. These amounts include any calcium that you get from your diet.

Be diligent about D. If you diligently slather on the sunscreen in summer or stay indoors all winter, you could be shielding yourself from the sun's vitamin D. If you fall into either of these categories, Dr. Schoenbeck insists that vitamin D supplementation is essential. Women who already have reduced bone density should get up to 800 IU of vitamin D daily.

Crank up the K. Keep eating dark leafy greens such as lettuce, broccoli, and spinach. Their high vitamin K content helps your body produce osteocalcin, a protein building block for bone.

Remember magnesium. Help your bones absorb calcium by getting this important mineral in foods like bananas and baked potatoes with skins. If eating a dozen potatoes is enough to drive you bananas, Dr. Schoenbeck recommends supplements of 500 milligrams a day. Many calcium supplements include magnesium, but if you take a combination supplement, be sure you are not exceeding 2,500 milligrams of calcium. Because this is a high amount of magnesium, you should check with your doctor before taking supplements if you have heart or kidney problems; also, supplemental magnesium may cause diarrhea in some people.

Hip, hip, ipriflavone! Derived from the isoflavone daidzein, found in soy, this supplement has been studied extensively in Japan, Italy, and Hungary, where it's used to prevent and treat osteoporosis. "Because it's synthesized, you really can't get it by eating soy," advises Dr. Schoenbeck, so ask your practitioner if it's an appropriate option for you.

Ipriflavone is really exciting, says Dr. Schoenbeck, because research indicates that it slows bone loss without the potential problems of estrogen. A dosage of 200 milligrams three times a day is her recommendation for women who shouldn't use hormone-replacement therapy or for those who do use it but want additional bone help. (If you can't find an ipriflavone product, look in the bone-health-supplement section of a health food store and read the labels to see if it's an ingredient.)

It's probably not a good idea to take isoflavone supplements instead of ipriflavone products, even if you're just taking a small amount of isoflavones. It looks like you get the most health benefits from eating whole soy foods, which have many other components in addition to isoflavones. The isoflavones seem to be very important but not the whole story, and if you take them in isolation from the other components in soy, they may even be harmful under some circumstances.

Extend your exercise. Take weight-bearing workouts a step further, advises Dr. Schoenbeck, with extension exercises like yoga and stretching to help maintain good posture.

Control Toxic Attacks: Liver Health

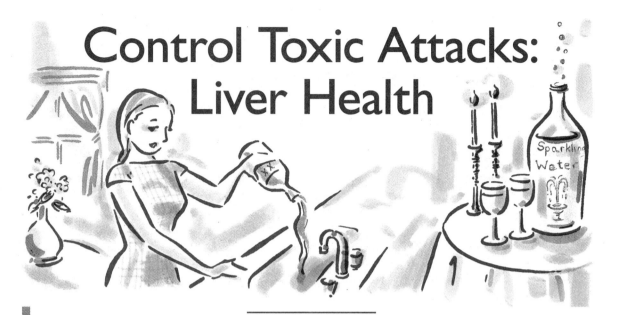

In December 1991, country singer Naomi Judd clung to the spotlight, clearly reluctant to leave the stage, following a farewell performance with her daughter Wynonna in Murfreesboro, Tennessee. At 45, she was being forced into retirement by a virus that attacked her liver and sapped her strength: hepatitis C.

"I was sometimes unable to get out of bed," Judd later wrote. "After a concert, I would literally fall onto my bed . . . in my stage outfit and high heels and fall into a deep sleep. No one had ever seen me even have a cold, so everybody around me knew something was wrong. . . . I knew so little about hepatitis. I didn't give it a second thought even though I'm a registered nurse."

Like Naomi Judd, few women suspect that they may be vulnerable to this vicious ailment.

"Many people used to think of liver disease as something that affected only alcoholics," says Melissa Palmer, M.D., a liver specialist in Plainview, New York, and author of *Dr. Melissa Palmer's Guide to Hepatitis and Liver Disease*. "Hepatitis is something that most folks don't really think about, but it's something they should definitely be aware of."

Why? Because unlike other internal organs, such as your stomach, your liver is essential to life. Its complex role in your body can't be taken over by other organs or replicated by machine. It takes nutrients from your blood and breaks them down into glycogen, the fuel that cells use to create energy. It converts drugs absorbed from your digestive tract into forms that are easier for your body to use. It detoxifies your blood and excretes substances that would otherwise be poisonous. It produces bile, a detergent your body needs to dissolve fat, and manufactures substances that help blood clot. Your liver also is a storage tank for certain vitamins, minerals, and sugars. So it's extremely important to do your best to keep your liver in peak condition.

Easily said, but here's the rub: If your liver is sick, you may not know it until it's too late. Even when as much as 70 percent of its tissue is damaged, you may not notice any symptoms that something is terribly wrong.

"The liver is a silent organ. Most of the time, it just does its job. It doesn't complain. It just keeps doing all of its many functions as best as it can even when it's sick," Dr. Palmer says.

So it's critical that you do all you can to prevent liver diseases, particularly hepatitis, an inflammation of the liver that afflicts at least three million American women.

Risk Factors

Although alcohol abuse, certain drugs, and herbal preparations can cause hepatitis, the majority of cases are triggered by viruses. The most prevalent ones in the United States are known as hepatitis A, B, and C.

Hepatitis A infects about 150,000 Americans each year and accounts for about 25 percent of all cases of hepatitis in this country. It's usually transmitted by consuming contaminated food or water. Cold cuts and sandwiches, fruits, vegetables, juices, milk and other dairy products, salads, shellfish, and iced drinks are frequently implicated in outbreaks of this form of hepatitis. It's occasionally passed on by infected restaurant workers.

Of the many strains of hepatitis, hepatitis A is the one you'll most likely encounter if you travel overseas, particularly to countries with lax sanitary conditions. Hepatitis A can also be transmitted by deep kissing, by having unprotected anal sex, and very rarely by using contaminated needles to administer intervenous drugs. Hepatitis A is seldom life-threatening—only about 100 people die from it each year—and 99 percent of those who get it usually recover within 6 months without serious complications.

About 5.7 million American women have been exposed to the hepatitis B virus. Hepatitis B is spread in infected blood and other bodily fluids. It can be acquired through sexual intercourse and sharing razors, needles, and toothbrushes with people who are carriers. Infected mothers can also pass it in their breast milk to newborn infants. The virus is also quite hardy. It can survive on a dry surface for up to 7 days and is 100 times more contagious than HIV, the virus that causes AIDS. Most adults who contract hepatitis B fend off the infection within a few months and develop an immunity that lasts a lifetime (but they remain susceptible to other viral forms of hepatitis). Up to 1 in 10 people who are infected with hepatitis B will develop chronic hepatitis, a persistent inflammation of the liver that lingers for more than 6 months and can be life-threatening. In fact, hepatitis B claims about 5,000 lives each year.

Hepatitis C is the most common form of viral hepatitis, accounting for 40 percent of all chronic liver disease, and is the leading reason for liver transplants in the United States. This virus, like hepatitis B, is a blood-borne disease. It is not spread by sneezing, coughing, hugging, or other forms of casual contact. About 1.2 million American women are infected with hepatitis C. Most of these women have experienced either no symptoms or only mild ones, and few realize they're carrying the virus.

A significant number of women contracted hepatitis C from blood transfusions prior to 1992, when screening tests were developed that dramatically lowered the risk of becoming infected with the virus from donated blood. In fact, the Centers for Disease Control and Prevention has not had a reported case of acute hepatitis C acquired through blood transfusion since 1994. Today, 60 percent of hepatitis C infections are acquired through sharing needles to inject drugs. Tattooing and body piercing are potential sources of transmission. Although hepatitis C can be transmitted sexually, the risk of infection is very low, especially if you are involved in a mutually monogamous relationship, Dr. Palmer says. About 20 to 30 percent of people who have hepatitis C develop cirrhosis (scarring) of the liver within 20 years. Cirrhosis can progress to liver failure or, in some cases, liver cancer.

Prevention

Prevention of hepatitis is mostly a matter of staying out of harm's way and using a bit of common sense. Here are a few practical tips that will help you dodge this nasty infection.

Scrub away. Practicing good hygiene may reduce your risk of contracting hepatitis A, says Marlyn Mayo, M.D., a liver specialist and assistant professor of internal medicine at the University of Texas Southwestern Medical Center at Dallas. In particular, be sure that you and your family members wash your hands after every visit to the bathroom and before meals.

Shelve raw shells. There may be more than a pearl hidden in a raw oyster, Dr. Palmer says. You may find hepatitis A lurking there as well. So if you enjoy shellfish, make sure that it's well-cooked.

Nab gamma globulin. If you suspect that you may have been exposed to hepatitis A, ask your doctor about getting a shot of gamma globulin. This blood product helps boost your immunity and, if taken within 14 days of exposure to hepatitis A, can greatly reduce your chances of getting the disease, Dr. Palmer says.

Get jabbed. Vaccines to prevent hepatitis A and B are available, and they are a wise precaution if you are at risk for either of these diseases, Dr. Palmer says. If you are traveling overseas, for instance, where the risk of hepatitis A is much greater than in this country, plan on getting the vaccine. And do it well in advance

NUTRITION: FUNDAMENTAL IN THE FIGHT AGAINST CHRONIC HEPATITIS

A well-balanced diet is essential in coping with chronic hepatitis B or C, says Heidi Gennaro, R.D., a registered dietitian and spokesperson for the American Dietetic Association.

"When people find out that they have hepatitis B or C, they want to do everything they can to help themselves. They usually become born-again health food nuts," she says. "They're almost looking for miracle foods or a miracle kind of diet plan. And there really isn't one except getting back to basics." Here's how Gennaro suggests you get started.

Ax alcohol. Even modest amounts of alcohol can have a toxic effect on your liver, particularly when you're trying to fend off a chronic disease. So if you have hepatitis, stop drinking right now.

Break bread. Breads, cereals, rice, and pastas, especially those made from whole grains, are loaded with B vitamins, fiber, minerals, and trace elements. In essence, these foods are your body's best fuel and can help keep you energized, particularly if you develop cirrhosis. Eat at least six servings a day. (A serving can be merely a slice of bread or bowl of cereal.)

Eat enough protein. Protein helps your body repair damaged liver tissue and produce new blood cells. At the earliest stages of chronic hepatitis, you need to consume 0.8 to 1 gram of protein and 25 to 35 calories for every 2.2 pounds of body weight. Check food labels for protein contents (they will be listed in grams). Meats, cheeses, milk, yogurt, tofu, nuts, and seeds are good sources of protein.

Strive for five. Eat at least five servings of fruits and vegetables daily. Not only are fruits like oranges and vegetables like broccoli loaded with vitamins and minerals, they're also a great source of antioxidants.

Shore up your inner reserves. A low-potency multivitamin-and-mineral supplement—one that contains no more than 100 percent of the Daily Value for any single nutrient—can complement a healthy diet by providing nutrients to keep your body functioning at optimum capacity.

of your trip because you'll need two doses, the first of which must be received at least 4 weeks before you leave the United States.

As for the hepatitis B vaccine, consider getting it if you are sexually active with more than one partner, share needles, or are a health-care worker. Hepatitis B vaccination is also required for newborns since the virus can be passed from mother to baby.

So far, there is no vaccine for hepatitis C.

Because the vaccines for hepatitis A and B are fairly new, doctors aren't certain how long they will be effective. But Dr. Palmer tells her patients that the vaccinations definitely will protect them up to 7 years, and possibly for a lifetime.

Don't pick up strangers. Hepatitis B and, to a lesser extent, hepatitis C, can be sexually transmitted, particularly if you have multiple partners, Dr. Mayo says. So if you're not sure of your partner's history or if you practice high-risk sex, be safe rather than sorry. Use a condom.

Shave your risk. Don't share intervenous needles, razors, toothbrushes, or other items used for oral or personal hygiene with anyone, Dr. Palmer says.

Likewise, be wary if you or a family member chooses to get a tattoo or body piercing.

"You should insist that the tattoo artist use a new needle on you," Dr. Palmer says. "A needle that has been used before might transmit both hepatitis B and C."

Curb the herbs. Although herbal remedies are undergoing a renaissance, some plant substances are toxic to the liver and can trigger hepatitis, Dr. Palmer says.

CIRRHOSIS: ALCOHOL ABUSE ISN'T THE ONLY CULPRIT

Cirrhosis and alcohol. The disease and the sight of a skid row bum are inseparable as far as some people are concerned. But the truth is that cirrhosis, the scarring of liver tissue, can affect any of us, even teetotalers.

Cirrhosis of the liver is a degenerative disease in which healthy cells are replaced by scar tissue. As this scar tissue builds up, bloodflow through your liver ebbs, causing further complications such as internal bleeding and fluid retention. Although most people associate cirrhosis with alcohol abuse, even social drinking (one or two drinks a day) can trigger this condition. Cirrhosis also can be caused by a number of other offenders including diabetes, malnutrition, hepatitis, and certain medications and environmental toxins.

"No matter what causes the liver to become inflamed, if the liver stays inflamed for a long period of time, it will eventually respond by making scar tissue. When you've developed enough scar tissue inside your liver, then it distorts the structure and function of the organ. That's when we call it cirrhosis," says Marlyn Mayo, M.D., a liver specialist and assistant professor of internal medicine at the University of Texas Southwestern Medical Center at Dallas.

Many people with mild cirrhosis have no symptoms and appear to be well for many years. Others are weak, have a poor appetite, and develop malnutrition, jaundice, itching, and a bloody cough. Cirrhosis is usually progressive, and it can lead to liver failure or liver cancer.

Keep in mind that many herbs may have harmful effects on the liver that have not yet been recognized. In any case, it's important to keep your doctor informed about any herbs you are taking, Dr. Palmer says.

Signs and Symptoms

The most common symptoms of viral hepatitis are fatigue, mild fever, muscle or joint

Some types of cirrhosis can be controlled with strict diets, diuretics, vitamins, and abstinence from alcohol. There is no cure, but liver transplants may help some people with advanced disease survive. More than 25,000 people die each year from cirrhosis, making it the seventh leading cause of death in the United States.

When cirrhosis is caused by alcohol, it's usually the result of a condition known as alcoholic liver disease. A common, preventable health problem, alcoholic liver disease is caused by long-term abuse of the drug. Symptoms usually depend on how long and how much a person drinks. But heavy drinkers can begin showing signs of this disease in their thirties or forties. In women, as little as 6½ ounces of wine, 13 ounces of beer, or 2 ounces of whiskey consumed daily can spark tremendous liver damage.

Alcoholic liver disease triggers three types of damage within the organ as it progresses. The first stage, known as fatty liver, causes enlargement of the organ and abdominal pain in the right upper quadrant of the belly. Alcoholic hepatitis, the second stage, is an acute illness often accompanied by nausea, vomiting, fever, and jaundice. In the final stage, alcoholic cirrhosis occurs, a condition that affects 10 to 15 percent of people who abuse booze.

The only treatment for alcoholic liver disease is to stop drinking. If that happens, the liver can repair some, but not all, of the damage done to it by alcohol abuse, and the person will likely live longer.

aches, nausea, vomiting, loss of appetite, vague abdominal pain, and, in some instances, diarrhea and weight loss. Some people notice dark urine and light-colored stools, followed by jaundice, in which the skin and whites of the eyes appear yellow. Itching of the skin may develop. But often, these symptoms are mild and can be misdiagnosed as a flu or another annoying but innocuous viral infection.

Just as frequently, hepatitis is an insidious disease that causes no outward symptoms for months or even years. This is particularly true of hepatitis B and C. In fact, up to 90 percent of people infected with hepatitis C show no symptoms until decades later when the virus's relentless assault on their livers shows up during medical tests. Some scientists suspect that in the early 21st century, the death rate from hepatitis C will triple or even quadruple to more than 24,000 people a year. In comparison, each year about 14,000 Americans die of AIDS-related conditions.

Don't Panic!

The symptoms for hepatitis are at best extremely vague. So it's possible that you really do just have a cold or a flu, says Dr. Mayo. Fatigue, loss of appetite, headaches, and other symptoms associated with the virus can also be signs of depression or thyroid problems, two conditions that often are easily treatable.

Even if it turns out that you do have hepatitis, there are plenty of other reasons not to panic. "There are many new drugs available that have been found to be very effective at eradicating the virus, and there are plenty of new therapies on the way," Dr. Palmer says.

Who Do I See?

See your family physician if you develop flu-like symptoms that persist for more than 2 weeks, jaundice, or any other signs of hepatitis. You also should seek care if you had a transfusion of blood, plasma, or other blood components before 1992 or have ever engaged in practices that might have exposed you to the virus, Dr. Mayo suggests.

"If you've had some questionable sexual encounters or if you experimented with intervenous drugs at some point in your life—even if it was many years ago and you feel healthy now—you probably should consult your family physician and get tested, particularly for hepatitis C because it's such a silent virus. All the evidence we have accumulated suggests that your best chance of getting rid of that virus is treating it as early as possible," Dr. Mayo says.

What Can I Expect?

Shock. Fear. Numbness. Bewilderment. These are all typical emotional reactions to a diagnosis of hepatitis. But as frightened and confused as you may be, it's important to stay as calm as possible and learn as much as you can about the specific type of hepatitis you have contracted, doctors say. Keep in mind that many people who get hepatitis don't fall into a high-risk category for the disease. You may not even remember how you were exposed to the virus—that's okay, most people don't. Instead, focus your energy on following your doctor's instructions, Dr. Palmer urges.

Physically, you may feel fine and not have any noticeable symptoms at all, or you may feel weak, drained, and run-down. In some cases, your body may fend off the infection in a few weeks and never cause you a problem again. In others, the infection may become a permanent part of your life.

WOMAN TO WOMAN

She Breathes Fire When the "Dragon" Roars

Elaine Moreland of McKinney, Texas, was a 32-year-old research-and-development analyst and the mother of two when she was diagnosed with hepatitis C in 1992. This is her story.

I have a dragon by the tail. It's not that I want to hold on to it. I have to. You see, I have hepatitis C, a viral infection that has caused havoc in my life for almost 20 years. If I let go, I know the dragon—that's what I call my disease—will swallow me whole.

So I hold on, day after day, refusing to give in.

I contracted hepatitis C in either 1977 or 1980, during the birth of one of my children. It was a routine practice back then to give women blood transfusions if they had cesarean births. And both of my deliveries were cesareans. What I didn't know at that time, and nobody else did either, is that there was this disease called hepatitis C that could be transmitted through infected blood products.

For the next decade, I felt progressively worse. I was exhausted all of the time, to the point that I couldn't find the energy to lift my arms and legs. It was as if they were made of lead. Finally, after years of being told by doctor after doctor that I was either a hypochondriac or depressed, I went to one physician and informed him that I wasn't going to leave his office until he found *something* wrong with me.

"There is a very individual response to this disease. In fact, one of the things that researchers are trying to figure out is why one person who gets exposed to a hepatitis virus gets acutely sick from the disease, while somebody else who gets infected with the same virus will be asymptomatic for 20 years before developing cirrhosis," Dr. Mayo says.

In either case, you may want to join a support

Conventional Wisdom

There is no specific treatment for hepatitis A other than getting plenty of rest. Hepatitis A does not cause chronic disease. In extremely rare cases, it can lead to rapid liver failure, but usually the infection will clear up in a few weeks or months, without complications. After you do recover, you will be immune to hepatitis A and never get it again.

Six months after infection is the key point in the course of hepatitis B and C. If you can eradicate these viruses from your body within that time, your chances of a full recovery without long-lasting harm to your liver are excellent, says Dr. Palmer. If, however, either of these viruses persists and you develop chronic hepatitis, as 10 percent of people who get B and 85 percent who contract C eventually do, then more aggressive treatment may be necessary. Both of these strains of hepatitis can be treated with interferon and other antiviral agents.

Great Alternatives

Anyone with a liver problem such as chronic hepatitis should consider taking milk thistle, says Andrew Weil, M.D., director of the program in integrative medicine at the University of Arizona College of Medicine in Tucson. This herb is nontoxic, and European research suggests that it stimulates regeneration of liver cells and protects them from toxic injury. Schisandra, a Chinese medicine, also helps the body heal chronic hepatitis. Both of these remedies have liver-regenerative properties.

Boy, did he find something wrong. When the doctor told me I had a disease that may require me to get a liver transplant, I freaked out. It's like having a terminal illness. There are no medical treatments that help everyone, and no cure yet, only holding on one day at a time.

And so that's what I do. The strange thing about hepatitis C is that sometimes it is like it is breathing fire, and you're just consumed with it. Other times, it is a very benevolent virus, and you don't even really know you have it. I really don't how I'm going to feel from one day to the next.

When I have what I call a bad dragon day, my mental capacities are severely limited (I call it a brain fog), and I'm not capable of making management decisions at that time. I also become very irritable and irrational on these bad days, which makes my family walk the outer limits around me. They say they put on their eggshell shoes.

The standard treatment for hepatitis C, interferon, isn't right for me. My doctor said I'm a nonresponder. Although there are other treatments that may help nonresponders, I made the decision not to undergo them. I was told that any further treatments with interferon could cause my virus to mutate into a more powerful form that would be resistant to future drugs. For now, I don't do much except take vitamins, experiment with a few herbal remedies, and have my doctor monitor me.

I simply don't let the virus rule my life. So I hang on and pray to God that someday I'll be able to slay this dragon. And you know, I think I will.

group to learn more about coping with your disease and any side effects of treatment such as nausea and diarrhea. For information about one in your area, check with your doctor or write to: the American Liver Foundation, 75 Maiden Lane, Suite 603, New York City, NY 10038-4826. Support groups are also available on the Internet at sites such as Hepatitis Neighborhood.

WOMEN ASK WHY

Why do I feel so lousy the next day after drinking just a little, when my husband drinks a lot and wakes up feeling great?

There are big differences in the way the bodies of men and women metabolize alcohol. A lot of it has to do with body mass. The average man weighs more than the average woman. Naturally, a larger body has to take in more alcohol before side effects begin to show up. The bigger you are, the harder it gets to become inebriated. But there's more to the story. Variations in a key enzyme called alcohol dehydrogenase, which helps break alcohol down into sugars in the stomach, may also contribute to a woman's susceptibility to alcohol. The differences may mean that we are exposed internally to the alcohol itself for longer periods, so we're more susceptible to its side effects. In short, we tend to get drunk more easily, and we take longer to get over any ill effects that liquor might cause, including a nasty hangover.

Expert consulted
Marlyn Mayo, M.D.
Assistant professor of internal medicine
University of Texas Southwestern Medical
*   Center*
.Dallas

"I have known a number of patients who have reversed hepatitis C using natural remedies like these," Dr. Weil says.

Milk thistle products (also called silybum or silymarin) are available in most health food stores, Dr. Weil says. Follow the dosage on the label. He prefers extracts standardized to contain 80 percent silymarin in tablet or capsule form. You can take milk thistle indefinitely, he says.

Together with milk thistle, take schisandra berries, the fruits of a Chinese medicinal plant, Dr. Weil advises. The dried berries look like red peppercorns and have a fruity, peppery taste. You can either eat them whole or, better yet, make them into a tea. Add 2 teaspoons of berries to a quart of cold water, bring to a boil, cover, lower the heat, and simmer for 20 to 30 minutes. Strain, and drink throughout the day. The berries may be difficult to find, so you may want to look for capsules of this herb at health food stores and follow product labels for dosages.

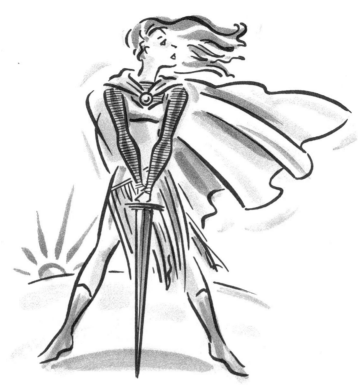

PART FOUR

A New Beginning

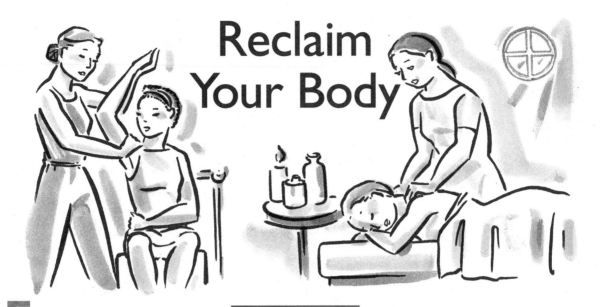

Reclaim Your Body

Fighting off an illness is difficult, exhausting work. And when the job is done, your body needs to rest and recover. It needs a vacation, so to speak. So if you could take your body anywhere, where would you go?

To a tropical paradise, lying under a palm tree and drinking chilled coconut milk from the shell, as aquamarine water laps quietly at the sand around your feet? To a mountain retreat in the deep stillness of the woods, where the only sounds are the chirping of birds and the occasional rustling of leaves as squirrels play among the branches? Or maybe to a spa, where the most taxing thing that happens all day is an hour-long massage followed by a visit to the sauna and jacuzzi?

Makes you feel better just thinking about it.

And that's the point. You don't need an island or a mountain or a spa. You can help your body recover after an illness through the medium of your mind, using techniques like meditation, guided visualization, or yoga. They're all part of complementary medicine, a branch of healing that often uses the mind-body approach to assist in the healing done by conventional medicine.

Good Complements

"Complementary medicine is a place where women can reconnect and reclaim their bodies. It really empowers a woman to reawaken her ability to care for herself," says Cynthia Knorr-Mulder, a licensed nurse practitioner and manager of the complementary medicine program at the Center for Health and Healing at Hackensack University Medical Center in New Jersey.

Here's a sampling of the many complementary therapies that can help you reclaim your body after a serious illness or accident.

Sit calmly. Meditation can help you reclaim your body and possibly speed healing after an illness or injury, Knorr-Mulder says. "Meditation relieves stress and decreases blood pressure, heart rate, and your perception of acute pain, while it increases your perception of health. Cumulatively, all of those things put you in a better position for healing," she adds.

Meditation has been shown to reduce high blood pressure, headaches, and chronic pain. In addition, studies have shown that it boosts the immune system. Some practitioners, such as Knorr-Mulder, also use it to help women cope with cancer and heart disease.

You can try a simple meditation technique yourself. Find a quiet spot and sit in a comfortable position. Take a few slow, deep breaths. As you breathe out, ask yourself, "Who am I?" Notice the associations that sprout in your mind: "I'm a wife," "I'm a mother," "I'm angry." Allow these thoughts to flow through your consciousness—enter and exit your brain—without judging them. If you find yourself thinking, "I'm a cancer survivor" and begin worrying about a recurrence or ways that the disease has affected your family, let those thoughts go and refocus your mind on the fundamental question, "Who am I?"

Try to practice this meditation twice daily for 15 to 20 minutes each session.

See yourself healthy. Your imagination can help you reclaim your body even after a major trauma, says Barbara Dossey, R.N., director of Holistic Nursing Consultants in Santa Fe, New Mexico, and author of *Florence Nightingale: Mystic, Visionary Healer.*

Imagery is the language that your mind uses to communicate with your body. Each day, thousands of thoughts, images, and sensations flit through your brain. At least half of these thoughts are negative even when you're healthy. If you've had a serious accident or illness, these negative thoughts may alter your

WOMAN TO WOMAN
She Used Physical Therapy to Recuperate after Her Cancer

An experienced oncology nurse, Marcy Fish, 43, of Wyncote, Pennsylvania, had spent much of her career caring for women with breast cancer. After she was diagnosed in 1998 with ductal carcinoma in situ (an early, noninvasive form of cancer) in her left breast, she had a mastectomy and breast reconstructive surgery. Her recovery from the surgeries went smoothly except for some range-of-motion problems in her left shoulder. Concerned, she consulted complementary-care specialists at Fox Chase Cancer Center in Philadelphia. Here's her story.

During reconstructive surgery, the plastic surgeon removes fat and muscle from the abdomen and uses it to form the new breast. So after the surgery, my breast area and underarm region had things attached where things didn't used to be attached. Plus, scar tissue formed from my lower abdomen all the way up to my left underarm. I received 2 months of physical therapy at the Complementary Care Center at Fox Chase, and they got me back to full range of motion. They were able to teach me stretches that would give me maximum benefit without any harm. A lot of it was a matter of regaining confidence in my body. I wanted to get on with my life, but I didn't want to hurt myself doing it.

After I finished physical therapy, I began taking dance classes that the center was offering to its patients. It is a way of continuing the exercises necessary to maintain your muscles' full range of motion but in a nonthreatening, noncompetitive way. We're not out there dancing to *Twist and Shout.* These dances are actually just very gentle movements set to music and specifically geared for people who have just undergone surgery.

I think physical therapy and dance have helped in a couple of ways. It's accomplishment without competition. I'm able to say, "Hey, I did that today." And there is the camaraderie that comes from people who are in the same situation. It's almost like a support group of sorts because all the women in the room know that all the others have been through a similar situation.

physiology, complicate your recovery, and possibly make you more susceptible to ongoing physical problems, such as arthritis or urinary tract infections.

On the other hand, if you harness positive images in your mind, you can help your body heal itself. In essence, your brain and body react to an imagined sensation as if it were a real one.

Here's how you might use guided imagery to help you reclaim your body after a heart attack, says Dossey. Set aside 20 minutes several times a day to practice. Resting in a comfortable position, take several deep breaths. Imagine that somewhere deep inside of you a brilliant light begins to shine. Allow the light to grow brighter and more intense. The light is powerful and penetrating. Notice that a beam begins to grow out of it. This beam shines into your body as you prepare to nurture your heart. Travel on this beam of light to your heart and just watch it for a few moments. As you observe your heart, clearly see all of its structures interacting in a coordinated, rhythmic dance. Listen to your heart beat. Hear it going stronger and stronger.

Next, imagine running your hands along the muscular walls of your heart, feeling the strength in them. If you've had a heart attack, spend some time observing the area of scar tissue. Notice how smooth and strong the scar is. See the new collateral blood vessels starting to form. Watch as these vessels bring blood, proteins, oxygen, and other substances to the healed area.

Spend a few moments seeing how you will look when your heart is completely healed. Imagine looking at yourself in a mirror. See yourself as strong, straight, and healthy. Visu-

REAL-LIFE SCENARIO

She's Afraid to Exercise Now That She Has Had a Silent Heart Attack

At 52, Fran was feeling great. She had her own small house-cleaning business, she was taking an aerobics class at night, and she had planned a cross-country trip with her husband. In fact, the only time she could remember being ill over the past year was on Super Bowl Sunday, when she had felt a little light-headed and had an upset stomach. During a routine physical, her family doctor told her that her blood pressure was too high and her heartbeat sounded a little irregular. He gave her an electrocardiogram. The result floored her. Apparently, she'd had a silent heart attack at some point and hadn't even realized it. The information so frightened her that her entire life went on hold. She quit her job, figuring it was too strenuous. She decided to postpone her trip because she didn't want to be on the road if an emergency occurred. And she decided to give up exercising altogether. Now, she does little more than sit at home, worry, and scan the Internet for information about cardiovascular disease. Does her life have to change so drastically?

Women tend to become depressed, withdrawn, and sedentary after heart attacks. In fact, after heart attacks, more women than men do not return to pre–heart attack levels of activity, particularly sexual activity, be-

alize yourself playing with friends or your family. Feel the strength returning to your lungs and your legs. Picture yourself being able to walk as far as you want, breathing easily and feeling robust.

When you have finished this guided imagery, take a few slow breaths as you regain awareness of your surroundings. Know that you are doing your best to help your body heal.

Yoga your way, I'll go mine. Yoga, a system of precise posture and breathing, can reduce levels of stress, relieve pain, promote wound healing, and improve your stamina and sense of well-being, whether you have a chronic illness, such as diabetes, or you're recovering from an

cause they are afraid of triggering additional cardiovascular events. So Fran's reaction is quite typical.

But no, she doesn't need to alter her lifestyle to such a great extent. She should ask her doctor for further testing such as a stress echocardiogram, an ultrasonic record of heart activity, in order to determine how well her cardiovascular system is working. Then, after being thoroughly evaluated by her cardiologist and receiving his approval, she should immediately enroll in a supervised cardiac-rehabilitation program. She should be encouraged to exercise and lead a normal life. With proper care, she should be able to lead a completely active life. In fact, Fran might have a better life than she led before because a heart attack, rather than limiting your life, often can serve as a wake-up call to make choices, such as dietary changes, that can enhance your whole being.

Expert consulted
Marianne Legato, M.D.
Founder and director
Partnership for Women's Health
Columbia University College of Physicians and
Surgeons
New York City

acute condition, such as a heart attack, says Cynthia Geesey, a Kripalu yoga instructor at the complementary medicine program of Fox Chase Cancer Center in Philadelphia.

Practitioners believe that moving your body into different poses forces blood out of vital organs, allowing fresh blood to take its place. This not only cleanses your organs but also provides more nutrients, making your organs stronger and more resistant to disease.

This ancient Indian practice has been used successfully in many cardiac-rehabilitation and cancer-treatment programs. "It's a gentle, compassionate modality that is able to work with the limits of your body at a given point in time. So if you have heart disease or have just undergone quadruple-bypass surgery, you can still do yoga," Geesey says.

And you can do it without twisting yourself into a pretzel, she says. To try it, stand as straight as possible with your back against a wall and your feet shoulder-width apart. Let your arms dangle at your sides. Inhale for a slow count of 10. As you do this, slowly raise your arms out to your sides and over your head. Then, exhale—again for a slow count of 10—and lower your arms back to your sides. Do this for 2 to 3 minutes twice daily.

There are many types of yoga, and it may take you some time to find a form that you feel comfortable doing. Phone around and talk to a number of instructors before committing to any classes, Geesey suggests. Talk to your doctor before starting a yoga program, and be up-front with instructors about any medical conditions.

Stretch your limits. Though they're often overlooked, occupational and physical therapies are potent allies that can help you reclaim your body when you have—or have had—cancer or heart disease, says Karen Mohr, a physical therapist and research director at the Kerlan-Jobe Orthopaedic Clinic in Los Angeles. If you feel fatigued as a result of your disease or treatment for your disease, a physical or occupational therapist can teach you energy-conservation techniques that will help you do household chores or other activities. If you have had extensive surgery that has left you with limited motion in your joints, weak muscles, or decreased endurance, a physical therapist can help you improve your range of motion and increase your strength and endurance. If you suspect that

THERAPEUTIC MASSAGE

Therapeutic massage is a terrific addition and complement to regular medical care that offers many benefits. It has been known to improve circulation and lymph flow, increase relaxation, and decrease stress and tension, says Caron M. Hunter, a licensed massage therapist and associate director of integrative pain medicine at ProHealth Care Associates in Lake Success, New York. Massage, when done by a medical professional, may help to promote recovery from the muscle fatigue and soreness that can result from exercise.

Many physicians now recommend using it on patients with acute or chronic pain because massage helps rid the muscles of lactic acid, a substance that can lead to body aches. Massage may also be used as a modality in heart disease because it reduces stress that can cause the blood vessels to narrow and the heart to work faster. If you are recovering from one of these diseases, however, you should discuss this option with your physician before receiving therapeutic massage. Other medical conditions, such as asthma, arthritis, sports injuries, gastrointestinal disorders, and muscle spasms, can be helped by frequent massage therapy.

You might wonder how getting a back rub is different from undergoing therapeutic massage. Many states have strict criteria and education requirements for training as a massage therapist. Massage therapists who graduate from accredited schools are medical professionals, and in many states they sit for licensing exams. They are trained in all aspects of the physical anatomy and have a deep understanding of appropriate application and proper technique for a variety of medical conditions. So while a back rub from a friend may be soothing and feel good, a treatment from a licensed professional will incorporate educated and proficient massage that not only soothes but also heals.

If you would like to find a reputable massage therapist in your area, write to the American Massage Therapy Association, 820 Davis Street, Suite 100, Evanston, IL 60201-4464.

you might benefit from either of these therapies, discuss it with your doctor.

Note: Your state or insurer may or may not require a referral from a doctor for you to see a physical or occupational therapist.

Feed Your Recovery

Making dietary changes is one of the most important things that you can do to reclaim your body after heart problems or cancer, says Nicole Napolitano, R.D., a certified dietitian-nutritionist and senior nutrition consultant at ProHealth Care Associates in Lake Success, New York. Here are some ways that you can use diet to help you regain your health.

Skip the fat. Of the eight controllable risk factors for heart disease, including elevated cholesterol and excessive weight, five have been linked to high-fat eating. Dietary fat may also have a role in 60 percent of cancers that affect women. Unfortunately, a typical American woman eats enough fat each week to equal six sticks of butter.

To keep your body healthy after you recover, start by limiting your fat consumption to no more than 25 percent of your total caloric intake, says Napolitano. The easiest way to control fat consumption is to count grams because that's how fats are measured on nutrition labels. So if you eat 1,500 calories a day, for instance, and want to keep your fat intake below 25 percent, multiply

1,500 by 25 percent. That's 375 calories. Then, divide that by 9, which is the number of fat calories in 1 gram of fat. Rounding off, you get 42, the number of grams—from all the foods that you eat in one day—that you can allocate for fat.

In particular, eat no more than 10 grams of saturated fat—usually found in red meats and other animal products—or products like mayonnaise and margarine that contain hydrogenated oils, says Napolitano. These fats increase the amount of the bad low-density lipoprotein (LDL) cholesterol and triglycerides in your arteries. One way to ensure that you stay on track is to eat no more than one palm-size, 3-ounce serving of lean animal protein daily. Experiment with miso, tofu, and other soy products. These alternatives are terrific substitutes for meat in your diet, and they contain substances that may lower your risk of recurrent cancer or heart disease.

Give three cheers for the superfoods. Eat at least eight servings of fruits and vegetables daily, Napolitano urges. Keep in mind that a serving can be as simple as eight baby carrots, ½ cup of cooked vegetables, or half of a banana. Make sure that your mix includes spinach, chard, romaine lettuce, and other green leafy vegetables. These foods provide plenty of folate and beta-carotene, which are loaded with an-

tioxidants that help fend off recurrences of heart disease and cancer.

Fruits and vegetables are also a source of fiber, which may help speed foods through your body so that fewer carcinogens can be absorbed by your digestive tract. In addition, dietary fiber may help lower blood cholesterol.

In general, you should eat four bites of fruits, vegetables, and whole grains for every bite of meat you take, says Napolitano.

Pitch a safety net. Supplements such as vitamins C and E and beta-carotene can promote recovery and reduce your risk of recurrence of heart disease or cancer, Napolitano says. These antioxidants prevent the formation of free radicals, rogue cells that can damage arteries and promote dangerous cellular mutations. Take 250 to 500 milligrams of vitamin C, 100 to 400 IU of vitamin E, and up to 6 milligrams of beta-carotene daily.

Go nuts. Some varieties of nuts and seeds are excellent sources of vitamin E, Napolitano says. They also contain the heart-healthy good kind of fat, monounsaturated fat. But keep in mind that they are chock-full of calories and should be used sparingly. Try adding a tablespoon of sunflower seeds to a salad or six almonds on a scoop of nonfat frozen yogurt.

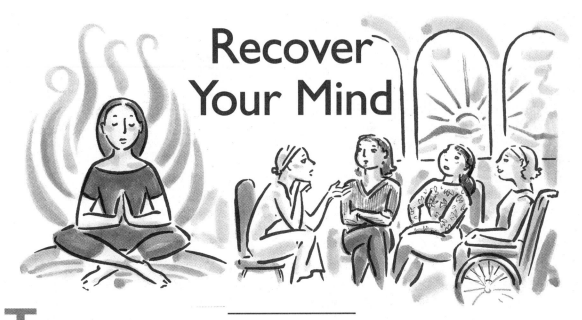

Recover Your Mind

The medications are gone. The treatments are finished. The illness is cured. And life continues. Except that living will never be quite the same now because you'll always know that catastrophe can strike again at any time, any place. You feel fragile, uneasy, and vulnerable. Surviving doesn't feel like a victory.

"Survivorship just means that you're alive. You're breathing," says Wendy S. Harpham, M.D., author of *After Cancer*. "It tells you nothing about the quality of your life or how you've integrated the disease experience into your outlook on life. People rid of their disease but paralyzed by untamed fear and anxiety or trapped by an inability to accept the loss of a body part or function are not healthy survivors."

Healthy survivorship after cancer, stroke, heart disease, and virtually every other catastrophic illness or injury depends as much on your mind-set, on your attitude, as it does on your medical care, Dr. Harpham says. And she should know. She has survived seven recurrences of non-Hodgkin's lymphoma in a decade.

Regaining a Healthy Mindset

Certainly, there are limits to what your mind can do for you. All the positive thinking in the world probably won't prevent a recurrence of cancer or another heart attack if your body harbors health-threatening changes. But the mind is a good place to start your quest for healthy survivorship, Dr. Harpham says. Because if you believe that you can make a difference, you're more likely to get the best medical treatments available, eat well, get regular exercise, and do other health-promoting activities. At the same time, regaining your mental vibrancy will help to quiet worries, douse fears and anxiety, and resist denial, all of which can prevent you from living a rewarding life.

"How do people become healthy survivors? By obtaining sound knowledge, finding and nourishing realistic hope, and acting effectively," Dr. Harpham says. Here are a few ways that you can tweak your mental outlook and become a healthy survivor.

Make knowledge your best friend. Healthy survivors realize that ignorance is not bliss, Dr. Harpham says. Learning all you can about your disease and its consequences may initially add to your anxiety. In the long term, however, basic medical knowledge tames fears and helps people regain a sense of control over their world. So gather all the information you can about your illness (or have a friend or family member do it if you can't for some reason). It will lessen your fears and at the same time allow you to recognize problems early, when they are most treatable.

Return to sender. Write a letter expressing how you feel about what has happened to you, suggests Anne Coscarelli, Ph.D., a psychologist and director of the Rhonda Fleming Mann Resource Center for Women with Cancer at UCLA Jonsson Cancer Center in Los Angeles. It can be cathartic. "Writing a letter gives you the freedom to express whatever it is you feel. And expressing those feelings—whether of anger or anxiety—helps you grieve, let go, and move forward," Dr. Coscarelli says. "You can write whatever you want as long as it embodies what you feel. Expressing yourself is an important part of the process."

Keep up the correspondence. Once you've completed that first letter, take out another sheet of paper or open a new file on your computer. Write a new letter to yourself that embraces who you are now. Don't be afraid to express love for yourself and to reaffirm that you're still the same wonderful person that you've always been. Write these letters to

yourself as often as needed. You don't need to show them to anyone. If you wish, you can throw them away after each session or keep them as a reminder of your journey.

MY MAMA TOLD ME
If I cross my eyes, can they really get stuck?

Of course not. Muscles surrounding your eyes allow you to move them in toward your nose to the crossed position. But they certainly won't get stuck there any more than bending at the elbow will cause your arm to get stuck in one position.

Normally, eye movement is coordinated so that both eyes look at a person or object at the same time. Eyes that cross involuntarily occur when this ability is disrupted for some reason. In most cases, crossed eyes result in double vision and should be immediately brought to your doctor's attention. In adults, crossed eyes can be triggered by diabetes, high blood pressure, brain injury, stroke, thyroid disease, or myasthenia gravis or other disorders of the muscles or nerves surrounding the eyes. Special glasses or surgery may be required to correct this problem in adults.

Infants under 3 months old may occasionally cross their eyes, and it is no cause for alarm because they are still learning how to coordinate their eye movements. But if it persists—and it is very important to be watchful for crossed eyes or lazy eye among young children—the lazy eye can weaken and lead to impaired vision.

The real myth is that a child with crossed eyes will outgrow it. This is a dangerous misconception. If a child is treated from ages 7 to 9, crossed eyes can usually be corrected without lingering problems. After that age, vision impairment becomes permanent. The earlier the detection of a possible disorder, the better.

Expert consulted
Sheri Rowen, M.D.
Assistant clinical professor of ophthalmology
University of Maryland School of Medicine
Baltimore

Bust a gut. Hilarity—sidesplitting laughter—can help you cope with your anxieties and fears during a major illness, Dr. Coscarelli says. It allows you to look at scary situations, such as checkups, in funny or sarcastic ways. Humor also is a distraction from the loss and suffering.

"Humor is life-affirming and life-giving," Dr. Coscarelli says. "When you laugh, you breathe deeply. So the harder you laugh, the more deeply you breathe, and the more you will relax."

Rejoice! Celebrate each year of survival as you would any important anniversary, Dr. Coscarelli suggests. It will help turn negative memories into positive ones.

"Make a point of letting others know that you're a survivor. Celebrate what you've accomplished in the past year and what you intend to do in the upcoming 365 days," she adds. Host a party, plan an adventurous trip, or simply invite a few friends over to share how wonderful it is to be alive. Your appreciation for life may teach others about living.

"Having people around you for these moments can be very helpful. It will allow you to talk about what you've gone through, acknowledge any sadness you may feel, and share a sense of pride in having survived. All of those things can be very comforting after a serious illness," Dr. Coscarelli says.

Cling to others. Many women participate in survivor groups after their disease, Dr. Coscarelli says.

"Once treatment stops, for any disease, you can suddenly feel alone in the big, scary world. There is a sense of isolation, of being detached.

REAL-LIFE SCENARIO

She Became a Real Hypochondriac after Her Melanoma Was Removed

Jeanine, 41, never thought much about her freckles. So far as she could remember, she'd always had them. Then, something happened. After a sunburn one summer, a dark brown freckle on top of her foot became very black and looked almost perfectly round, almost like a burnt match head. She paid it no mind until she heard a dermatologist talking about black moles and melanomas on a television talk show. That pricked her attention. She immediately made an appointment to see a doctor and, within a few days, had the mole removed for tests. She almost went crazy with anxiety waiting for the results. Fortunately, the tests were negative. But the doctor told her that the mole was a "precancerous, dysplastic nevus" and that she would have to keep an eye on her moles from then on. Without meaning to, he had badly frightened her. From that day on, she found herself checking her moles so diligently that she spent most of her time in front of mirrors or under a magnifying glass. And she goes back to the doctor almost monthly to question him about something on her skin. She can't go on living this way. What should she do?

Jeanine does have an increased risk for melanoma because of her light, freckled skin and history of dysplastic nevus. She will always have a higher risk of developing melanoma than the average person. But her overall risk is still quite low. Jeanine can influence her overall chance of developing skin cancer, too. First of all, her risk of developing melanoma can be decreased if she avoids sun exposure, uses sunscreen every time she goes into the sunlight,

So who understands and can share the feelings you have about the changes that have occurred in your life? People who have been through the experience. That's why survivor groups can be so helpful. They bridge the gap," Dr. Coscarelli says. Ask your medical team about survivor groups in your area.

Don't fear the Reaper. At some time. you

and wears clothing that protects her skin when she is outdoors (such as wearing a T-shirt over her bathing suit when she is not swimming).

She can also decrease her risk of death from melanoma through appropriate screening, including regular, but not obsessive, head-to-toe inspections of her skin as well as an examination by a dermatologist every 3 to 6 months, or as often as her doctor recommends. Jeanine would probably benefit emotionally from regular visits because of her anxiety. If she does see something suspicious during one of those checks, certainly she should notify her doctor right away and not wait for her routine scheduled visit.

If Jeanine is examining herself regularly and has good checkups with her doctor, continued fearfulness is counterproductive. It isn't decreasing her risk of cancer. It's simply taking away from her quality of life. She needs to tame that fear. A good starting point would be for her to realize that she can still protect herself from this cancer without obsessing about it. She should understand that the chances of her developing a life-threatening melanoma in a month or two are almost zero. She should continue to do skin self-exams every 1 to 2 months (or however often her dermatologist recommends). If she doesn't find anything during her skin exam, she has to trust that she is fine. Also, she has to trust that because she is being diligent, if she should develop melanoma, she will probably pick it up early, when it has a good chance of being curable.

Expert consulted
Wendy S. Harpham, M.D.
Author of After Cancer

may hear or read that someone you know has died of the same disease you had. It can be frightening and sad. You may feel a shiver down your spine because it rattles your sense of being safe from death, Dr. Harpham says.

You can rein in your fears if you remember that the other person's death has no effect whatsoever on what will happen to you. Keep in mind that there are many factors that affect any individual's chances of long-term survival from an injury or disease. Look for ways in which your disease's course differs from that of the person who has passed away, suggests Dr. Coscarelli.

Dr. Harpham suggests reaching out to others and talking about your feelings. It's okay to cry and feel sorrowful. Paradoxically, this grieving can actually affirm your will to live, help you embrace a positive attitude, and enhance the quality of your life.

If reading obituaries disturbs you, skip that page of the newspaper. If you find yourself dwelling on obituaries and you cannot stop thinking about death, seek professional help to sort out your fears and feelings, Dr. Harpham suggests.

Watch your mouth. Language is powerful. Wordplay is not trivial mental gymnastics, it is one of the forces that shapes our perception of reality, Dr. Harpham says.

"I did an interview on a national news program a few years ago that identified me as 'Wendy Harpham, cancer victim.' I cringe when I hear those words," she says. "Victims, by definition, feel helpless and hopeless. Survivors have succeeded against a challenge or threat. I have always considered myself a cancer survivor. Sometimes, I'm a cancer patient. But I have never been a cancer victim. Cancer victims and cancer survivors are in the same situation, but they have different frames of mind."

So whenever you catch yourself using negative language, stop and change your thinking. If necessary, jot down a new, more positive phrase. Dr.

WOMEN ASK WHY

If medicine can treat depression, why do I need to see a counselor?

Depression must be treated with a multifaceted approach because it has many aspects. Some are biochemical and can be relieved by medication. Others are situational and can't be treated with drugs. You need behavioral tools to help you through those moments. That's why counseling, in conjunction with medication, is so important.

Medication is just one tool. It's not going to help you understand what has happened to you. And it's not going to help you find other ways in which you may be able to deal with your feelings. If you're relying solely on medication and your disease happens to recur, you will probably be at a disadvantage compared to others who have gone through counseling and learned additional coping skills. Finally, medication alone won't help you move beyond what has happened to you or give you greater understanding of where you want to go and who you want to be now that you're recovering.

Expert consulted
Anne Coscarelli, Ph.D.
Director
Rhonda Fleming Mann Resource Center
for Women with Cancer
UCLA Jonsson Cancer Center
Los Angeles

books for both children and adults about coping with cancer.

Stop your mind from wandering. If you frequently find yourself ruminating on how you might deal with your disease if it recurs, stop. It probably won't help you. Set limits. If you find yourself drifting into an ugly scenario, do whatever you can to distract yourself. Be grateful for today and let go of worries about tomorrow.

"If a recurrence happens, I'll deal with it then," Dr. Harpham says. "I don't want to deal with it twice—now in imagination and again when it really happens."

Shrink it down to size. Don't be afraid to seek professional assistance, particularly if you have any of the following symptoms.

- You have a sad, worried, or empty feeling that never goes away.
- You think of suicide.
- You can't sleep, you're sleeping too much, or you're waking too early in the morning.
- You have trouble concentrating or making decisions.
- You feel as if you can't get back into the swing of life, even though your illness has long since passed.

"Just because you seek professional assistance doesn't mean that there is something terribly wrong with you," Dr. Coscarelli says. "It's just part of the experience, and it may be helpful to talk to someone who can help you sort these feelings out and build an effective emotional toolbox that will make it easier for you to cope with them in the future."

Harpham, for instance, never thinks of her cancer as incurable, even though there are no known cures for it today. Instead, she describes her disease as one of the types of cancer for which scientists are still looking for a cure.

Chart a new course. Instead of letting an emotion such as anger or anxiety fester, use it as a positive force to change other lives. Some women have created Web sites on the Internet that are loaded with information about their diseases. Others become advocates, fund-raisers, or volunteers. Dr. Harpham has written several

Revive Your Spirit

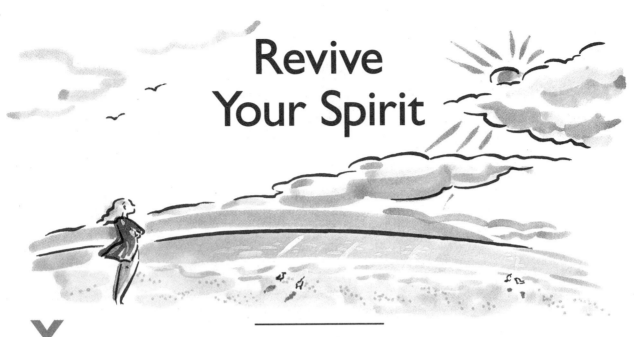

You shake a fist at God and ask, "Why me?"

That's how many of us react to getting sick. Finding meaning and nobility in your situation is probably the furthest thing from your mind, at least initially. But meaning and nobility are there.

After living with illness for a while, many women, out of necessity, slow down and take stock of their lives, says Rabbi Nancy Flam of Northampton, Massachusetts, director of the spirituality institute Metivta, based in Los Angeles. "They make priorities in terms of what's most important, and often that turns out to be love and wisdom. They might have preferred to come to those decisions in a more pleasant fashion, but people can certainly change their lives for the better because of serious illness."

That's not to say that suffering is a good thing, of course. "I have known only a handful of people who would claim that they wouldn't have traded their cancer for good health because of what they learned and how they grew as a result of having it," Rabbi Flam adds. "But I've met many, many more who felt that they would rather have remained healthy and shallow.'"

The point is to make the best out of a less-than-wonderful situation. With some effort, you can turn sickness into an opportunity for real spiritual renewal.

What Does It All Mean?

Pain and adversity can make you bitter, or they can make you better. It's your choice, says Freda Crew, D. Min. (doctor of ministry), director of Truth for Living Ministries in Spartanburg, South Carolina, and author of *Get Off Your Own Back*. "I tell people, 'It's here, it's a reality, you can't deny it. So let's get everything we can out of it.'" Here are some ways in which you can begin to do that.

Change the "Why me?" to "What am I going to learn from this?" It can take some time, but you can change from feeling like a helpless victim to regaining a sense of control in your life. Just ask yourself, "If this is part of my life's journey and lesson, what am I going to get out of it?" says Rabbi Judith Abrams, Ph.D., coauthor of *Illness and Health in the Jewish Tradition.* "This is more useful than wallowing in your situation."

Seek the truth. "Very often, pain and adversity will cause a sincere person to start yearning for answers," says Dr. Crew. "But the truth doesn't usually end up laid on our doorsteps. The best way to find answers is to become a searcher, a seeker after truth and reality, and then to deal with things as they really are."

For instance, Dr. Crew says, you're kidding yourself if you think that by trying to please God you'll avoid pain or suffering during your lifetime. "The Bible, which we turn to for our truth, never says such a thing. We have conjured this up ourselves," she says. Realizing that God is not to blame, that you are not to blame, that you are not being punished, and that suffering is pretty much a fact of life for everyone can make a big difference in helping you cope with your illness.

Turn to prayer. Most religions have prayers that you can say when faced with anxiety, such as "The Lord is my shepherd" (Psalm 23). And many have prayers for the morning and evening. "These are natural times in the day when one realizes that one is living on a globe, spinning through the cosmos, affected by the sun and gravitational pull," Rabbi Flam says. "When the light changes, it is really an opening and awakening of our awareness. It's also a time when one realizes that everything changes, that everything is fleeting, transient, momentary, and so it is really a time for becoming aware of the moment and its blessings."

Instead of asking, listen. "I strongly believe that prayer is about listening and waiting for a

WOMAN TO WOMAN
From Here to Eternity

Joann May, 43, an administrative assistant from Philadelphia, had never considered herself a particularly religious person. Then one evening, when she was 37, her heart stopped during an asthma attack. Before the night was over, she would forever change her concept of God, heaven, and life on Earth. Here's her story.

I was at home, folding laundry, not feeling so great, when my chest started to tighten, and I knew I was in trouble. I took some of my usual inhaler, but it didn't work. My last resort, which I had never used before, was an EpiPen, a shot of epinephrine, which is a hormone sometimes called adrenaline. That didn't kick in either, so I called my dad, who lived a few blocks away, and told him I needed to go to the hospital. I remember going down the first five steps to the car, and that's it. I collapsed out in the street, and the paramedics worked on me there for close to an hour. My heart stopped once in the ambulance and twice more in the hospital, so I was pretty much going in and out of it for about 5 hours before I woke up on a respirator in the hospital.

It's very hard to explain what happened to me during that time, because it was like a dream, a beautiful dream. I was very disappointed that it started to fade so quickly after I woke up.

I did move through a tunnel toward a point of light, which I

response—not asking for a response the way I want it, but listening for what is the right thing to do, which may be something I never even thought about," says Sister Felicia Petruziello, a licensed professional clinical counselor at St. Joseph Wellness Center in Cleveland. "Part of prayer is learning to listen my own heart, my own gut." People do better in adversity if they realize that they do have some control in the matter. "So they need to recognize that there are answers for their situations but that the answers

learned is common during near-death experiences. I had a spiritual guide who gave me a tour of the universe, and that was a sense of the vastness of the universe, of being there at its creation, of being a part of the universe from its beginnings. I had no sense of self; I was everything and everything was me, including God. It was a very reassuring feeling, and I felt very safe and protected. I felt unconditional love and joy and peace.

I didn't want to go back into my body. I started arguing with God, and God said that I needed to go back because my mission here wasn't complete. I was told that I hadn't loved enough and that part of my mission was to spread the message to love one another.

I never had much of a sense of God, but now I know that he is not some guy with a beard who sits on a throne and says who's in and who's out.

My sense now of "heaven," of the afterlife, is that what happens to you when you die is your choice. You can choose to exist in a state of unconditional love, or not, and it all comes from how you forgive yourself for the blunders that you made in your life. You totally judge yourself. You feel the pain that you created during your life, and it all comes back to you as its creator. When you forgive yourself, you experience the love, joy, and peace to move on.

I am not afraid of death now—no way. But I don't do anything to risk my life. I know that's not the way to get back there. I was told that I wouldn't be going back there any time soon.

might not be immediate or apparent. There are answers if we wait and listen," she says.

The Most Important Job You'll Ever Have

Illness often motivates women to start looking for the places where their lives have gone off course. "Just realizing where you need to do some work and then starting in on it can

help resolve a lot of unhealthy stress," Dr. Crew says. Here are some ways you can do that.

Explore where your life may be out of balance spiritually. Now is your chance to restore that balance. Are you working too hard? Feeling sorry for yourself? Unable to accept others' comfort? Unable to experience joy or wonder? Carrying around feelings of fear, guilt, anger, or shame?

"We need to take an inventory of our lives, to take a journey into our very thoughts, motives, relationships, and behavior," Dr. Crew says. "Are there those we have failed to forgive, or do we have unresolved conflicts with people? Are we breaking God's law and unwilling to stop?"

Count your blessings. Learning to shift your attention from what is gone or painful to what you have and enjoy can help you cultivate a more positive attitude, says Sister Felicia. Some easy ways to cultivate a sense of gratitude are to say thank you to people and to God and say grace over meals. Take time to do things that you enjoy, to be a part of nature, and to realize that you are a part of something greater than yourself. Keep reminders of love and beauty around you—photos of loved ones, mementos of good times, a rock from a beautiful lake, flowers from your garden.

Pick up a Good Book. Words can convey hope and provide guidance, says Sister Felicia. "I frequently refer people to the Psalms because they are about feelings. I tell people that, often, when they are angry or distressed, that is their prayer. Sometimes, just yelling at God or crying out to God is your prayer, and the Psalms are very much that."

The Power of Prayer

If you think that praying is something you do out of helplessness when there's nothing else you can do, that you're simply humoring yourself, then you're underestimating its power. Studies, some of them controlled enough to qualify as scientific, suggest that prayer can have an impact on the course of an illness.

In one landmark study, patients in a cardiac-care unit were randomly divided into two groups. The members of one group were remembered in what's called intercessory prayer, prayers offered to help others, while the other patients were not prayed for. Neither the patients nor the hospital staff knew which patients belonged to which group.

The people doing the praying did it outside the hospital, using only the patient's first name, diagnosis, and general condition. They prayed for the patient's rapid recovery and freedom from complications.

Those patients who were prayed for had less congestive heart failure (8 versus 20), needed less antibiotic therapy (3 versus 17), had fewer episodes of pneumonia (3 versus 13), and had fewer cardiac arrests (3 versus 14). Twenty-seven of those in the group of patients who were prayed for did poorly while 44 of the others had a poor recovery.

A similar, more recent study, done with AIDS patients, found that healing messages sent from healers of both religious and secular traditions lessened the severity of the patients' illnesses and improved one measure of mood.

As for meditation, it's surprisingly well-documented for its ability to reduce blood pressure, relieve pain, and lower anxiety. In one study of people treated at the University of Massachusetts Medical Center in Amherst, those who meditated were able to use less pain medication and said that their pain was much less likely to stop them from doing things than people did who did not meditate. The meditators also reported less anxiety and depression.

In another study, psoriasis patients who meditated while undergoing ultraviolet light treatment had their skin clear up significantly faster than did nonmeditators.

The Book of Job also does a good job of presenting anguish and introspection in the face of adversity, Dr. Crew says.

Ask others to pray for you, and listen to what they say. A powerful feeling of being loved can come from knowing that people are praying for you. "I have a real sense that I am being covered in prayer, and as I gain strength, I realize that people's prayers are being answered," Dr. Crew says.

Most religions have special prayers for healing body and soul. In Catholicism, it's the Anointing of the Sick; in Judaism, it's the Mi Shebarakh.

"Praying publicly for someone who is sick has a double effect," Rabbi Flam says. "There is the prayer one offers up or within, which provides hope of healing body and soul. And there is the connection that the community makes around the person who is ill. The person's name is said and everyone is informed, so there are also visits and food and offers to help."

Make meditation a habit. Meditation has proven abilities to calm and center you, to slow your breathing, and to lower your blood pressure. To do a simple meditation, just close your eyes and pay attention to your breathing, Rabbi Abrams suggests. Focus on a short phrase, perhaps a verse from the Bible or a spiritual picture or scene. "Just focus and allow yourself to stay in that state for a while," she says. "It doesn't have to be hours. Even if all you do is a minute, you will feel yourself calm down, and pretty soon all it takes for you to begin is to focus on your breathing and the calming will start. You develop a reflex."

Start treating your body like the temple that it is. Whether it's overeating, drugs, or alcohol, if you are having trouble overcoming bad habits and addictions that are contributing to your health problems, pray for help, Sister Felicia advises. "If we ask for anything in our religion, it is for strength. And even though we believe that God is always with us, there is something comforting about the request."

Seek spiritual companionship and renewal. Lots of people start reattending church or synagogue, even after an absence of many years, because of sickness or some other crisis. And that's nothing to feel ashamed or embarrassed about, Dr. Crew says. Studies show that people who attend religious services regularly are healthier and live longer.

"In fact, you might want to look for a church that ministers to people in need, to people who are hurting," she says. "Check out what kind of support system they have for people who are going through crisis. Who is there to assure them that they are loved and cared for? Are people encouraged to reach out to others? Are others often willing to help if they know about a situation or are asked to help?"

Take the disheartened into your heart. "People who help others always seem to say, 'I

MY MAMA TOLD ME

Will sitting too close to the television really wreck my eyesight?

Scientific research has proven Mom wrong on this one. Studies that look at the number of hours children spend watching TV have been unable to find any link with vision problems, she says. It's true that long hours of close vision work, such as reading, are associated with nearsightedness. But nearsightedness has never been linked with TV viewing. You can sit right on top of the TV, and it doesn't seem to matter.

On the other hand, a fair number of people develop eyestrain—fatigue or aching around and above the eyes—from viewing a computer screen for long hours. And they may be more likely to have such problems as they get older and need bifocals. The solution is a special pair of glasses designed just for computer work. The lens targets your "middle vision" at about 24 inches. In the old days, we used to call these piano glasses. They were prescribed for ladies who played the piano and needed to be able to read the music.

Expert consulted
Karla Zadnik, O.D., Ph.D.
Associate professor in the College of Optometry
Ohio State University
Columbus

get more out of this than the people I am helping,' and I feel that way myself," Sister Felicia says. "I am amazed at what people can get through, and I believe we gain strength from going outside of ourselves to help others."

"People feel a deep impulse to redeem some of their suffering by helping other people," Rabbi Flam adds. "Instead of letting their suffering be an event of disillusion and destruction, they salvage their experience and make meaning and build up the world again by providing a comfort and a sense of compassion and wisdom and guidance for others."

Say the "D" Word

It's the elephant in the middle of the room that nobody talks about. While we fear pain and suffering, we also mourn the eventuality of our own deaths. Instead of ignoring it, it's better to ponder it and come to some terms with it, spiritual leaders say.

Confront your mortality. Are you afraid of dying? Most people are, and they resist thinking about it, Dr. Crew says. "But I don't know of anything that makes us face mortality more

quickly than a serious illness or accident. People have to start thinking about what they believe, and they start working through the grief of their own death."

Create your own immortality. Whatever your sense of life after death, there are ways that you can leave an impression of yourself here, Rabbi Abrams says. "Whether you're a car mechanic or a college professor, strive from your heart to pass on your special knowledge, and you'll make the most of the gift you have been given. Give to your family, friends, your community, to anyone to whom you can act as a parent. Do good deeds, and know that your good deeds live on after you, that the world is a better place for your having been here."

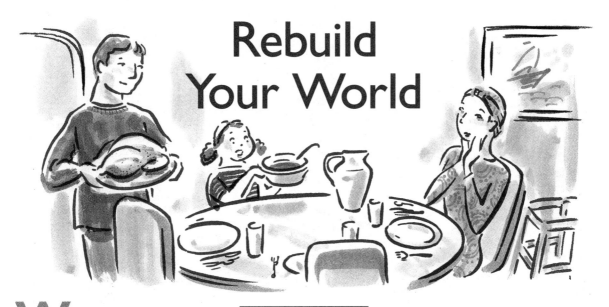

Rebuild Your World

When Linda McCartney phoned her husband to tell him that she'd been diagnosed with breast cancer, he dropped everything and rushed home to be with her. For the next 2½ years, as they fought her disease, he gave her unstinting support and devotion. Even in her final moments, he was at her side whispering love and encouragement to her.

It's a beautiful story, and we all hope that, should we ever get sick, our loved ones will be as loyal and caring as Paul McCartney was. Unfortunately, we know that life—and people—don't always turn out as we'd hoped.

Illness sometimes brings out the best in people, but not always. "It can really draw people closer together, but it also has the potential to blow a relationship apart," says Catherine Classen, Ph.D., a clinical psychologist at Stanford University School of Medicine.

Being sick can make us very needy, and the constant challenge of meeting our needs can leave our partners feeling resentful and inadequate. A husband accustomed to being waited on at home, for example, may suddenly find his new role as caregiver too much to handle.

"Illness can be the stress that finally ends a troubled relationship," says Mary K. Hughes, R.N., a psychiatric clinical nurse specialist at the University of Texas M. D. Anderson Cancer Center in Houston. "Husbands *do* leave—not always, of course, but often enough that it isn't a rare occurrence. And when it happens, it's devastating to a woman."

On the other hand, a couple that survives an illness often uses the challenge to put trivial problems into perspective and to come to appreciate and value each other more than ever. "It's about both sides being gentle with each other and knowing that illness, acute or chronic, is really hard to process into a relationship," says Susan Brace, R.N., Ph.D., a clinical psychologist practicing in Los Angeles. "Both people are likely to feel as if life is being changed and it isn't fair—life *is* being changed, and it *isn't* fair."

When Opportunity Knocks

What may seem especially unfair is that, even when she's ill, a woman often remains the emotional caretaker of her family, if only because no one else will assume the role. But what at first looks like a burden can turn into an opportunity to strengthen the relationships she cares about most, if she takes a few simple steps.

Give the gift of time. Head off resentment by encouraging family members to take some time for themselves, Dr. Classen says. "I'm not saying that they need your permission, but they feel less guilty if you tell them something like 'I'm okay here for a while. Why don't you go to a movie or take some time to yourself?'"

Show appreciation. Don't take your family for granted. Every day, let each of them know how much they are appreciated and valued, says Mary Cerreto, Ph.D., an industry consultant and specialist in relationships and illness in Natick, Massachusetts. "We forget to praise or reward the little things we have come to expect, and the people who do the most get the least thanks sometimes." Don't assume that those who are helping you know you're grateful for what they do. Tell them.

Be explicit. The more clearly you can express your needs, the more likely you are to have those needs met, Dr. Classen says. "A lot of women say how disappointed they are in a particular family member's response. Often, these women have a wish that they can't bring themselves to ask for explicitly. But if they don't ask, they don't get. So they need to state their wants and needs very clearly."

Deal with feelings. To keep the lines of communication open and your relationships strong, you need to discuss whatever emotions you and your family may be going through concerning your illness. But don't stop there. "Recognizing feelings without moving ahead is

---

REAL-LIFE SCENARIO
She's a Real Do-It-Yourselfer

April, 45, would call herself a self-reliant woman. She cooks, she cleans, she repairs her house, and she has raised four kids on her own—her husband, a merchant marine, had been at sea most of the time. When she became a widow 6 years ago, she went out and got herself a job cashiering at a local drugstore and worked weekends cleaning offices for a local transportation company. Then, this breast thing happened. It started with a lump in her right breast, and before she knew it, she was in the hospital recuperating from a mastectomy. Her sons and daughters instantly showed up to help, offering to cook and clean for her and to help her financially, but she's finding it difficult to accept their kindness. She somehow feels ashamed of being off her feet for a while, and, as a result, she's been irritable and cranky with everyone. As much as her kids want to help her, they're starting to resent the way she treats them—and she knows it. But she just can't help herself. What should she do?

At some emotional level, April is probably convinced that she doesn't deserve any help, and she doesn't want to be a burden to others. In fact, if she hasn't been so nice to be around lately, there's a good chance that it's because she feels guilty about accepting help.

But why should she feel unworthy or guilty? After all, April has almost certainly given her children lots of care whenever they've needed it in the past, and now they're

---

useless," says Dr. Cerreto. "At some point, you have to say, 'Okay, now what do we do about these feelings?'"

For a son who is feeling neglected, for instance, you might say something like, "Now that Dad can't take you to baseball games as much as he used to, I've noticed that you've been getting angry at me more often. I can understand why. My being sick has really made some big changes in your life. What can we do about it?"

Or for a husband who has shut down and stopped communicating, you could say, "You've

eager to help her in return. By turning them away, she's robbing them of the opportunity to show her in concrete ways that they care about her and appreciate what she has given to them over the years. She may not realize how much doing things herself isolates her from her family.

April surely has chores or errands that other people could do to make her life easier right now: running for sundries, cutting the grass, cleaning the house, even doing some of the cooking. And by giving her children specific suggestions, she'll remain in control so that they don't go overboard and start trying to run her life.

As for financial help, if her pride won't let her accept money outright, her children can make the situation easier by offering to do things like fill her gas tank or pay for her groceries. If she still says no, they should be sensitive enough to accept her answer at face value.

April could benefit from easing up on herself. There may be days when the pain or stress of illness makes her irritable. On those days, it would help if she just let her children know that. A generous thank-you would make both April and those who care about her feel a lot better.

Expert consulted
Mary Cerreto, Ph.D.
Industry consultant and specialist in relationships and illness
Natick, Massachusetts

been so quiet lately that I don't know what you're thinking. I can't tell if you're worried, but I know you're sad. I'm sad, too. What can we do to start talking about it? I want to help you understand what I'm feeling and going through with this illness so that you don't worry so much and so that we can handle it together."

Bring Friends into the Fold

Friends react to illness as they do to any other difficult situation. "Some will be a wonderful example of what it means to be a friend, and others will feel helpless and not want to be there," says Dr. Brace. Close friends may have more presence of mind than even family members about what needs to be done and how you're feeling. Others will want to help but may be uncomfortable and unsure of how to go about it. Here are some ways you can help your friends support you.

Reach out and touch someone. Friends don't call for a variety of reasons. Your illness may have struck too close to home for them, they may lack confidence in their worth as companions during this time, or they may prefer to say nothing rather than risk saying the wrong thing. Their absence does not necessarily mean that they no longer care about you. You, too, may have withdrawn during part of your illness to protect your own feelings. But you can't draw comfort from an empty room.

If you really don't want to lose someone's friendship and you believe discomfort rather than fear is keeping a particular friend away, try a phone call to dissolve the barrier, Hughes says. And try using humor to break through the initial awkwardness. Tell a joke, laugh together, then say something like, "It feels so good to laugh. I haven't laughed in a while."

If you've been withdrawn because you were depressed, your closest friends should know. Your honesty will promote intimacy. But you don't need to tell everyone you know. To acquaintances, you might just say, "I wasn't feeling well," and leave it at that.

Help friends to help. Believe it or not, most people are grateful if there is something concrete that they can do to show their continuing

My Mama Told Me

Will swimming too soon after eating really give me cramps?

It's true that you are more likely to develop a side stitch, a muscle cramp in your diaphragm, if you do any kind of vigorous exercise soon after eating a large meal. And a cramp may make it difficult to swim since you're likely to want to curl up in a ball. But it's more uncomfortable than dangerous.

The cramp occurs because blood-rich oxygen is being diverted away from your muscles to your intestines to aid in digestion. Oxygen-deprived muscles can cramp up.

So that old "mom's rule" of waiting an hour after you eat before you swim laps isn't such a bad idea. Wait until you feel comfortable, until your stomach is no longer full. But feel free to get into the pool to just cool off or swim slowly. That shouldn't cause cramps, even with a full belly.

Expert consulted
Jane Katz, Ed.D.
Professor of health and physical education
City University of New York, John Jay College of Criminal Justice
World masters swimming champion
Author of Swimming for Total Fitness

Use friends as rehab helpers. Use their visits to structure your day. For instance, if your doctor wants you to start walking to rebuild your strength, have a friend take a walk with you, Dr. Brace says. Don't just rely upon going to physical therapy three times a week.

Learn to share. One of your best immediate resources is someone who has the same condition as you do and is doing well, Dr. Cerreto says. You may be able to find such a person in a support group, which can provide understanding, support, and companionship for both you and your family. Ask your doctor about local support groups, or contact American Self-Help Clearinghouse, St. Clare's Hospital, 25 Pocono Road, Denville, NJ 07834-2995. They will provide, free of charge, information on a support group nearest you. Or look in your local library for a copy of the book *The Self-Help Sourcebook, 6th edition*, which includes contacts for hundreds of groups. As you recover, sharing your experiences with others can help you regain strength and courage.

Work Things Out at Work

When you return to work, coworkers, like friends, will respond in a variety of ways. So you may need to deal with people individually. Some won't even know about your illness, and that's just as well, Dr. Cerreto says. "If you don't want to tell them, just say, 'I was sick. I was in the hospital, but now I'm feeling fine.'" But in some

friendship. So if a friend says, "Is there anything I can do?" take her literally. If you could use it, ask for simple assistance—to run an errand, to prepare a meal, or simply to come and visit. "These small acts bring friends back into contact and help them feel useful and needed," Hughes says. "You have done them and yourself a favor."

Assign a point person. Sometimes, one close friend can become the go-between for you and other friends, setting up visits from people, getting old friends back in the room, and calling people to tell them how you're doing, Dr. Brace says.

cases, it's good to have one cool, calm person around who knows what you have and who can help you if you need it.

If your illness has left you permanently disabled, you should contact your company's personnel office when you return to work. By federal law, the Americans with Disabilities Act requires employers of a workforce of 15 or more to make reasonable changes in your work site that will allow you to do your job, such as giving you a wheelchair-accessible work area.

If you're worried about not being able to get back up to speed right away, your employer may need to make some accommodations for you. Here again, you have legal rights.

On the other hand, if you're being coddled at home, returning to a situation where others do not think of you as sick may be the greatest therapy yet devised.

The Gift of Wisdom

When God said to Solomon, "Ask what I shall give thee," Solomon begged for wisdom. If you've recovered from an illness, or if you're still sick but you've learned how to cope successfully, you've received the very same gift, whether or not you realize it.

How so? From your own experience, you now know things about weathering illness that you never before realized. You know about the needs, the fears, and the wishes that being sick can create. You can use your newfound wisdom in

WOMEN ASK WHY

Why were people afraid to touch me when I was sick, even though I wasn't contagious?

Lots of people worry about getting or giving germs when they're around someone who is sick, even when the chances of transmission are slim. They know that some germs can be transmitted through touch, but they don't know enough to know when that's not likely to happen. And some people may worry about how touching might be received. They don't want to do something that might be taken the wrong way or that might cause pain.

What's more, people often don't realize how beneficial a caring touch is to someone who is sick. The love and comfort that is conveyed through touching often has benefits that outweigh the risks.

When you are visiting a sick friend, wash your hands before you have direct contact with her, especially if you are in a hospital and have been touching handrails and doorknobs. Then, try gently squeezing her hand during a conversation or laying your hand on her shoulder. If your friend squeezes back, smiles, or lays her hand over yours, your touch is welcome.

Expert consulted
Charlotte Eliopoulos, R.N., Ph.D.
Specialist in holistic geriatric and chronic-care
nursing
Author of Integrating Conventional and
Alternative Therapies

your day-to-day dealings with anyone who may be facing a challenge to her health. Here are some examples.

State the obvious. People who are sick or who have recently been sick often have trouble talking about what is going on for them, Dr. Classen says. "They may be afraid and kind of deny it," she says. "Or they may not want to burden one another with their own concerns. They may find that when they do try to talk about their worries, they don't get the response they want, and that's very painful, so they shut down." If someone is depressed, she may isolate herself all the more.

To break the ice, approach her directly. Just say, "What's going on today? You look sad," suggests Hughes. "That person is just waiting for someone to notice that she is different, that something is wrong."

People who have been seriously ill are often fearful of dying, of always feeling bad, of never getting well, of not knowing what's next. "Just getting these feelings out in the open and talking about them takes away some of their power,"

Hughes says. Someone who is depressed, however, may also need medication to be able to shake some of the oppressive feelings.

Be absolutely honest. Sick people just know things about their state of health whether the doctor tells them or not, Dr. Brace says. "Some people will say they're afraid that, if they're honest, they're going to hurt someone's feelings. But if you're honest, you at least have a real solid bridge to the other person, and if it hurts her feelings, you can apologize. If you're not honest, you have no bridge. And sick people feel most isolated not having those bridges. What makes the sick person feel most isolated is pretense, by the doctor or by the family. Sick people don't want to be lied to."

Index

Boldface page references indicate illustrations. <u>Underscored</u> page references indicate boxed text.